DATE DUE

Demco, Inc. 38-293

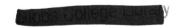

NEW ENGLAND INSTITUTE OF TECHNOLOGY
LIBRARY

Mental Health and Violent Youth
A Developmental/Lifecourse Perspective

Denise Paquette Boots

LFB Scholarly Publishing LLC
New York 2008

Library of Congress Cataloging-in-Publication Data

Boots, Denise Paquette, 1970-
  Mental health and violent youth : a developmental/lifecourse
perspective / Denise Paquette Boots.
     p. cm. -- (Criminal justice : recent scholarship)
  Includes bibliographical references and index.
  ISBN 978-1-59332-231-1 (alk. paper)
  1. Problem youth--Pennsylvania--Pittsburgh--Longitudinal studies. 2.
Problem youth--Mental health--Pennsylvania--Pittsburgh--Longitudinal
studies. 3. Violence in adolescence--Pennsylvania--Pittsburgh--
Longitudinal studies. I. Title.
  RJ506.P63B66 2008
  362.2'70974886--dc22

2007038019

ISBN 9781593322311

Printed on acid-free 250-year-life paper.

Manufactured in the United States of America.

Table of Contents

Acknowledgements

This monograph is the culmination of approximately four years of research and would not have been possible without the help of many talented people. First, my sincerest thanks to Dr. Rolf Loeber for allowing me the opportunity to work with such rich and meaningful data. Your mentoring and enthusiasm has been a great inspiration for me over the years. I am also indebted to Dr. Dustin Pardini and Ms. Rebecca Stallings, each of whom gave me great data support and insight into this complex dataset and all those syntax challenges along the way. I also wish to thank several other senior scholars who gave me valuable critiques and guidance throughout this project, including Dr. Kathleen Heide, Dr. John Cochran, and Dr. Richard Dembo. Special thanks also to Dr. Jennifer Wareham, who was always available for discussions about this project and various considerations. I want to express my gratitude to my colleagues at the University of Texas at Dallas who have offered encouragement along the way, including: Drs. Jim Marquart, John Worrall, Joylynn Reed, and Brian Berry. Finally, special thanks to Nancy Paquette for all her critical feedback, proofreading expertise, and unconditional moral support throughout every stage of this work.

Preface

Concern about violence, and especially violence perpetrated by our youth, is of great international concern currently. Newspapers, magazines, television interest programs, and talk shows highlight the prevalence rates of violence perpetuated by youth (along with violence perpetuated against youth) and the public at large is left to wring their hands and lock their doors.

Thankfully, Dr. Boots has conducted a study that not only helps us understand where we have been in the world of violent youth but also where we should go from here. Too often studies are conducted in what seems to be the vacuum of an ivory tower, where there are a lot of statistically significant findings but where there are few real-world implications. Luckily, Dr. Boots' work has clear ramifications for social policy in order to decrease the risk of, and perhaps even prevent the occurrence of, violence perpetuated by youth.

The study is symbolic of the best that real-world research has to offer. The data set is incredible and the original work by Rolf Loeber and Magda Stouthamer-Loeber and colleagues sets the stage for the newest line of findings related to violent youth. Unlike so many other studies that can be summarized by saying that "Most of the subjects were white and middle class" (Graham, 1992), this study is diverse in terms of participants' race/ethnicity, family socioeconomic status, and living circumstances.

The design of the study is also to be admired, given the focus on prospective, longitudinal work over the lifespan of youth in at-risk situations. In addition, the focus on dimensional as well as categorical conceptualizations of children's and adolescents' functioning is considered state-of-the-art in research on developmental psychopathology (Achenbach, 2005a). The use of well-established, psychometrically sound measurement instruments is a clear strength of the study, as is the use of multiple informants. The different findings from parent-reports versus teacher-reports highlights the need to gather information from a number of important informants in the lives of youth (Achenbach, 2005).

Dr. Boots' use of a developmental lifecourse perspective is consistent with the finest lines of research currently available and this perspective is crucial to the understanding of violence within youth and families (Caspi, 2000). By carrying on in a tradition that emphasizes the need for compassion, understanding, and firm consequences to youth who are violent, Dr. Boots has assembled a thorough, comprehensive, and interesting study that points to the connections between mental health problems in youth and their ultimate use of violence.

The work is interdisciplinary and should be of interest to scholars and students in the fields of criminology, psychology, social work, counseling, and public health. The study also has ramifications to work in genetics, behavioral genetics, environmental issues, family research, and educational foundations of the well-being of youth.

In the study of violent youth, there are often difficulties in combining data from divergent fields, partly because different subsets of youth are used in different arenas of investigation. For example, research on developmental psychopathology and within the realm of clinical child psychology has focused on youth who meet criteria for conduct disorder, whereas the tradition in research on criminology has been to define youth based on their status as juvenile delinquents (Frick, Stickle, Dandreaux, Farrell, & Kimonis, 2005). The current research seeks to bridge this gap by focusing on what the youth do rather than on a potentially arbitrary diagnosis or juvenile justice label. Thus, this work will hopefully bring researchers from divergent fields together with a common goal of finding ways to prevent youth from perpetuating violence.

The practical policy implications of these findings are tremendous. Although the results are not quite as consistent as might have been expected, there appear to be clear connections between psychological problems at certain points in the lives of boys and their ultimate level of severe violence. From a preventive perspective, one wonders how many acts of severe violence might have been prevented if some of these boys had received effective psychological interventions for their mental health problems before their ultimate usage of severe violence. Perhaps this book is one step in the direction of helping youth before they harm others and themselves in a way that is irreparable. Dr. Boots has shown us the path and has laid the ground work, so it is now up to us to put these findings into action in order to prevent more harm from and against the youth of today.

-- Vicky Phares, Ph.D.
Professor and Director of Clinical Training
Department of Psychology
University of South Florida, Tampa

CHAPTER 1

Violence and Chronic Offending as a Social Phenomenon

As a social problem, few garner more consistent attention in the media than violent crime. "In cities, suburban areas, and even small towns, Americans are fearful and concerned that violence has permeated the fabric and degraded the quality of their lives...violent deaths and incidents that result in lesser injuries are sources of chronic fear and a high level of concern with the seeming inability of public authorities to prevent them" (Reiss & Roth, 1993, p. 1). This fascination and enduring interest has generated an enormous body of literature, both scholarly and popular, which explores the etiology, perpetuation, and consequences of lethal and non-lethal forms of interpersonal violence.

Violence affects individuals, families, communities, and societies as a whole. Indeed, the public and the intellectual community of academia worldwide recognize the significant economic, medical, social, and psychological costs of violence. Security and safety are fleeting desires today for people living in urban centers plagued by violence and poverty (Kiser, 2006). The popular portrayal of violence, particularly in the media, as an important social problem in the United States consistently ensures that citizen fear of violent crime will be a top concern of Americans in public opinion polls nationally (Gallup Poll Online, 2003). Certainly, "when citizens are afraid of crime, it is life-threatening, personal violence that dominates their attention" (Zimring & Hawkins, 1997, pp. 11-12). Although public perception seems to indicate that Americans are afraid of being a victim of serious violent crime, the question remains to what extent violence is a serious problem in American society today. The present study is concerned with violence as it applies to individual criminal and antisocial behaviors.

Specifically, this work is designed to investigate whether the onset of childhood or adolescent mental health disorders may play a significant role in the development of later violent behavior and the continuance of serious antisocial acts over the lifespan. According to one recent study regarding mental health, most disorders begin in childhood and early adolescence though they may not be formally diagnosed and treated until much later in life (Patel, Flisher, Hetrick, & McGorry, 2007). The term "violence" is an ambiguous term that is used broadly across various temporal, situational, spatial, and structural contexts. Violence is defined, for the purposes of the present study, as "behavior by persons against persons that intentionally threatens, attempts, or actually inflicts physical harm" (Reiss & Roth, 1993, p. 35). Hereafter, violent and/or aggressive behaviors are discussed as they relate to situational contexts where such actions are almost always considered antisocial and are legally condemned by the criminal justice system (e.g., homicide, attempted homicide, rape, aggravated assault, robbery).

Other key terms also used within this paper include antisocial or deviant acts, delinquent behaviors, and youth violence. The terms *antisocial* and *deviant acts* refer to certain behaviors that break societal norms. Antisocial behaviors specifically refer to "acts that maximize a person's immediate personal gain through inflicting pain or loss on others" (Loeber, 1982, p. 1432). Both delinquent behaviors and youth violence are used herein to refer to behaviors of persons that are considered to be juveniles, or persons less than 18 years of age. *Delinquent behaviors* are defined broadly here to include any actions considered criminal (or illegal) for adults, as well as certain prohibited behaviors for minors that are status offenses due to age (e.g., smoking, truancy, curfews, underage drinking, sexual intercourse, etc.). *Youth violence* refers to intentionally harmful behaviors that seek to inflict harm on others and which are committed by individuals under age 18. Both "juvenile or minority status is determined on the basis of age and is a legislative decision" (Heide, 1999, p. 5).

There is a critical need to better understand the etiology of violent behaviors as they develop across the lifecourse. It is a well-established fact that the majority of violent adult offenders begin their criminal careers as youngsters. Accordingly, the necessity of identifying the causes and correlates of delinquency and violence in youths is obvious to academics and laymen alike. .

Violence in American Society

A large body of empirical literature has explored the prominence of violence historically in American culture (Brown, 1979; McGrath, 1984; Gurr, 1990; Butterfield, 1996; Lane, 1997; Kurtz, 1999). Widespread interest has focused in particular on increases in violence that occurred beginning in the 1960s (U.S. President's Commission on Law Enforcement and Administration of Justice, 1967). Zimring and Hawkins (1997) analyzed index crimes (offenses ranging from homicide to theft) in the U.S. for the years 1961 through 1980. The authors found a three-fold increase in the rate of index crimes through the 1960s and 1970s. Additionally, lethal violence more than doubled during the same period and extended into the 1980s, with 4.8/100,000 homicides recorded in 1960 and 10.2/100,000 recorded in the year 1980.

Violent crime peaked in the early 1990s. A steady decline in violent offenses began and continued into the year 2000 (U.S Department of Justice, Federal Bureau of Investigation, 1984-2002). Indeed, "violent crimes as recorded by the police dropped in 2000 for the ninth consecutive year, representing the longest-running decline in violent crime since the Federal Bureau of Investigation began keeping records in 1960" (Barak, 2003, p. 21). This trend continued in 2001 and 2002, with rates of 5.6 per 100,000 (Fox & Zawitz, 2004). These data come in stark contrast to previous levels of homicide in the U.S. in the early 1990s, with rates of over 10 persons per 100,000 being killed during the early part of this decade (Barak, 2003).

Alarmingly, the most recent Uniform Crime Reports (UCR) report on violent crime shows a renewed spike in serious offending throughout the nation. A preliminary report released in June 2007 indicated a 1.3 percent increase of violent crime when compared to 2005 rates (U.S. Department of Justice, Federal Bureau of Investigation, 2007). Interestingly, the most significant increases in violent offenses were located in relatively small towns (25,000-49,000 population) and medium-sized urban cities with a population between 250,000 and 499,999 inhabitants. These findings highlight the continuing struggle to ameliorate violence across the varied American social landscape.

A deconstruction of violent crime rates over the past several decades reveals that both adult and juvenile violence have emerged as a collective community problem. Beginning in the 1950s and over the next 40 years, violent crime rose over 600 percent, with juveniles accounting for the greatest increase in these numbers (Skogan, 1989). The coinciding rise of official reports of juveniles committing interpersonal acts of violence, beginning in the 1980s and continuing on into the 1990s, underscored the need to look at the youth violence phenomenon independently (Heide, 1992; 1995; 1999; Heide & Boots, 2003). This recognition of teen violence and aggression as a social and public health crisis, coupled with high-profile media accounts of school shootings in various settings across the country, led to the U.S. Surgeon General in 2001 to call for an investigation of the continuing issues surrounding youth violence in America. Following an exhaustive review of empirical and scholarly evidence on this problem, the Surgeon General stated, "there is a powerful consensus that youth violence is, indeed, our Nation's problem, and not merely a problem of cities, or of the isolated rural regions, or any single segment of our society" (U.S. Department of Health and Human Services, 2001, p. vi).

Youth Violence in America

The participation of youths in violent behaviors is not a new phenomenon. Rather, it is one that has had a significant historical precedent in the United States (U.S. Department of Health and Human Services, 2001). Indeed, some of the earliest literature that originated from the Chicago School found a relationship between youth violence and gang membership (Reidel & Welsh, 2002). A review of the FBI Uniform Crime Report (UCR) data shows a rise in juvenile crime rates beginning in the late 1980s and peaking in the mid 1990s (Heide, 1999). During the ten-year period between 1983 and 1993, arrests of violent youthful offenders increased an alarming 70 percent. Furthermore, the number of juveniles arrested for homicide surged three-fold for the same period (U.S. Department of Health and Human Services, 2001).

Additional analyses of UCR and National Crime Victimization Survey (NCVS) data by Cook and Laub (2002) showed a doubling of violent crime arrests for teenagers between the ages of 13 and 17. Their analysis found a stable arrest rate between 1975 and 1984. Data from the mid 1980s through the mid 1990s, however, indicated a two-fold increase in violent youth arrests. Since 1994, rates of juvenile violent arrests have fallen between three and six percent annually; in the year 2000, rates were comparable to those rates in 1984.

Further analyses of the juvenile arrest trends have shown that the majority of these arrests are for aggravated assault and robbery. For 2001 UCR data, approximately 94% of all violent arrests (approximately 63,000) were for these two offenses (Snyder, 2003). Of all arrestees, urban males, particularly minorities, are overrepresented for all young offenders reported as arrested in UCR data. Of particular concern are recent national self-report data from U.S. high school seniors. These data suggest that the rates of violent youthful offending, while falling from the highs of the 1990s, remain unsatisfactorily elevated for crimes such as robbery and assaults (U.S. Department of Health and Human Services, 2001).

With respect to homicide, the most lethal form of interpersonal violence, a review of UCR data provided by the FBI indicates that the number of teen homicide arrestees rose from just over 1000 youngsters in 1984 to over 3100 youths in the year 1994 (see Heide, 1999 for illustration; U.S. Department of Justice, Federal Bureau of Investigation, 1984-2002). For the decade between 1984 and 1993, juveniles accounted for 11.6 percent of all homicide arrests nationally; for the following decade between 1993 and 2002, youths accounted for an average mean of 14 percent of all homicide arrests. Since 1998, less than 1000 youths a year have been arrested for homicide offenses. These numbers are dramatically lower than those seen in the mid 1990s and are at levels not seen since the early 1980s. Despite these reductions in the number and rates of youths committing lethal violence, however, 2002 UCR data indicate that juveniles still account for approximately one out of every ten homicide arrests (9.6%) in the U.S. These 2002 homicide rates, at 7.3 percent, are still over two percent higher than 1984 levels.

Although chronic youthful violent offending is relatively rare (Klein, 1995; Esbensen, 2004; Loeber &

Farrington, 1998; Loeber & Farrington, 2000) and the majority of juvenile offenders desist from criminal activities in their early to mid 20s (Moffitt, 1993; Moffitt, Caspi, Dickson, Silva, & Stanton, 1996), boys, gang members, and youngsters of color continue to both engage and become victims of violent and antisocial behaviors in alarming numbers (Spergel, 1990; Moone, 1994; Thornberry, 1998; Jenson & Howard, 1999). There is evidence that there is a gap between when serious offending behaviors begin and when youthful offenders may be formally arrested and enter the criminal justice system (Elliott, 1994). Some studies have estimated that only five percent of serious violent offenders had official arrests as a juvenile despite years of violent acts against others (Howell, Krisberg, & Jones, 1995). Other studies have reported that upwards of 84 percent of serious violent offenders are never arrested for their crimes (Dunford & Elliott, 1984). Using National Youth Survey (NYS) data, Elliott and his colleagues have reported that nearly half of children who committed their first violent act prior to age 11 continued committing serious violence into young adulthood. Seriously violent careers began in these youths at age 12, doubling between the ages 13 and 14, peaking around age 16 and then dropping by 50 percent by age 18 (Elliott, Huizinga, & Morse, 1986; Elliott, 1994).

The first cohort studies to focus on chronic criminal offenders came from the seminal works of Wolfgang and his colleagues (Wolfgang, Figlio, & Sellin, 1972; Tracy, Wolfgang, & Figlio, 1985; Wolfgang, Thornberry, & Figlio, 1987; Tracy, Wolfgang, & Figlio, 1990) and West and Farrington (Farrington & West, 1990; 1993; West, 1969; 1982; West & Farrington, 1973; 1977). In his 1945 cohort study on "chronic offenders" in Philadelphia with five or more police contacts, Wolfgang and his fellow researchers found that these six percent of the cohort and 18 percent of all delinquent youths committed almost 2/3 of all violent offenses and 51 percent of total offenses (Wolfgang et al., 1972). In another study on the 1958

Philadelphia cohort by Tracy et al. (1990), seven percent of the cohort and 23 percent of all offenders were responsible for over 61 percent of the crimes, including homicides (60%), rapes (75%) and robberies (73%). Similar findings were reported in a cohort study by Snyder (1988) of juveniles in Arizona and Utah, with close to 2/3 of all murders, rapes, assaults, and robberies committed by 16 percent of all delinquent offenders.

There is some disagreement regarding what the appropriate number of violent offenses should be to be considered "chronic" offenders. Estimates have ranged from two to four serious assaults annually (Cohen, 1986), three or more (Loeber, Farrington, & Waschbusch, 2001), to six or more times (Blumstein, Farrington, & Moitra, 1985). Regardless of the number, a substantial body of research has suggested that the amount of crime committed by such chronic youthful offenders is disproportionate, increasing, and posing a serious public policy problem to society (Conduct Problems Prevention Research Group, 2002).

These earlier cohort studies are further supported by the work conducted in the U.S. Department of Justice Office of Juvenile Justice and Delinquency Prevention's Causes and Correlates of Juvenile Delinquency Program (see Thornberry, Huizinga, & Loeber, 1995; Loeber & Farrington, 1998; Thornberry, 1998). These data from three longitudinal, prospective study sites in Pittsburgh, Pennsylvania, Denver, Colorado, and Rochester, New York also indicate a high prevalence of violent offending by urban at-risk youths. In each of the three samples, between 14 and 17 percent of the youths were chronic, serious male or female offenders. These youngsters committed an astonishing 75 to 82 percent of all violent offenses committed by the samples (Thornberry et al., 1995). These results were consistent with previous studies, finding that only 6 to 14 percent of chronic violent persons were ever arrested for their violent crimes (Huizinga, Esbensen, & Weiher, 1996; Elliott, 2000).

These findings have been replicated in other studies and demonstrate that a very small number of troubled youths appear to be committing the majority of serious and violent crimes during childhood and adolescence (Farrington & West, 1993; Moffitt, 199a, Moffitt et al, 1996; Conduct Problems Prevention Research Group, 2002). Moreover, despite the apparent decline in official crime rates from past highs, self-reported youth violence has remained quite stable over the course of the past two decades (Jenson & Howard, 1999; U.S. Department of Health and Human Services, 2001). Consequently, "both self-reports and arrest rates for aggravated assault point to an ongoing problem of youth violence after the apparent end of the violence epidemic. Thus, the rise and fall in arrest rates for most violent offenses is set against more enduring rates of violent behavior" (U.S. Department of Health and Human Services, 2001, p. 27). What is less clear is how, and if, society should try to identify chronic offenders and intervene early in the lifecourse given that the majority of juvenile offenders do not commit serious crime and it is very difficult to predict the onset of persistent violent behaviors (Hamparian, Schuster, Dinitz, & Conrad, 1978; Strasberg, 1978; Howell et al., 1995). Such discussions frequently turn to the empirical evidence regarding developmental indicators of criminality and the impressive body of work that has been generated over the past two decades by lifecourse researchers.

Developmental Perspectives on Violence

It can be said that the study of violence as a social phenomenon is a multidisciplinary "collection of knowledge about criminal action, including psychology, sociology, psychiatry, anthropology, biology, neurology, political science, and economics" (Bartol & Bartol, 2005, p. 5). The driving theoretical force of the current study involves developmental explanations of deviant behavior subsumed under a general framework of mental health.

That is, a sizeable body of literature suggests that youths with poor mental health outcomes will be substantially more likely to have poor outcomes across life. What is more uncertain is which of the possible disorders will be significant at different points of childhood and adolescence, and whether different types of mental health problems will lead to different types of aberrant criminal behaviors.

This larger framework is loosely grounded in developmental criminology. Such developmental or "lifecourse" orientations have become increasingly prominent and popular in psychological and criminological circles as a heuristic framework to explain antisocial and violent behaviors over the lifespan (Loeber & Farrington, 1998). "Criminologists who employ a life-course perspective are concerned with identifying the processes whereby childhood disruptive behavior escalates to delinquency and crime, and with discovering the factors that enable some antisocial children to assume a more conventional lifestyle during adolescence" (Simons, Johnson, Conger, & Elder, 1998, p. 221).

Developmental psychopathological studies are a relatively new area of study, with the field largely developing in the 1970s. Despite the fact that much time and effort has been spent by an increasing number of researchers and clinicians on issues surrounding developmental normalcy versus dysfunction, there is certainly much still not understood about the mind and disorders of infancy, childhood, and adolescence. A number of studies have been designed in an attempt to better understand the prevalence and incidence of psychopathology at various stages in the lifecourse, including those disorders that emerge typically in the young.

While a truly comprehensive review of this large body of literature on developmental and lifecourse theories is not feasible here, perusal of these works indicates many influential contributors across a variety of lifecourse frameworks and methodologies. Researchers such as Elder

(1979; 1985), Loeber and Farrington (Loeber, 1982; Loeber et al., 1998; Loeber & Farrington, 1998; 2000; Fabio et al., 2006), Sampson and Laub (1990; 1993; 1994; Laub, Nagin, & Sampson, 1998; Laub & Sampson, 2003), Benson (2002), Patterson (1982; 1986; Patterson, De Baryshe, & Ramsey, 1989), Moffitt and colleagues (1990; 1993; Moffitt, Caspi, Rutter, & Silva, 2001; Moffitt, Caspi, Harrington, & Milne, 2002), Piquero and Mazerolle (Mazerolle, Brame, Paternoster, Piquero, & Dean, 2000; Piquero & Mazerolle, 2001; Piquero, Brame, Mazerolle, & Haapanen, 2002), and Tracy and Kempf-Leonard (Kempf, 1988; Tracy & Kempf-Leonard, 1996; Kempf-Leonard, Tracy, & Howell, 2001) for instance, have produced a convincing body of evidence regarding the advantages of using lifecourse theories. Several of these works suggest that serious, chronic offenders begin their antisocial behaviors in childhood and continue on these deviant trajectories throughout their lives, albeit it with opportunities along these pathways to desist in antisocial behaviors (see, e.g., Sampson & Laub, 1990; Loeber & Farrington, 1998).

These works suggest that the existence of early childhood behavioral problems is not enough to guarantee stability of dysfunction over the lifecourse and throughout adulthood. Simons et al. (1998), for example, reported that boys who had oppositional and conduct disorders in childhood were no more likely than healthy children to exhibit conduct problems during adolescence once they experienced improved parenting, increased school commitment, and separation from delinquent peers. Similar questions regarding the etiology and persistence of violent behaviors drive the present study, as well. A number of national and local studies point toward the co-occurrence of violent behaviors with other problem behaviors (Huizinga & Jakob-Chen, 1998; Tolan & Gorman-Smith, 1998). "However, by no means all serious violent offenders or even all chronic violent youths have co-occurring problems. Moreover, not all youths with problem behaviors are seriously violent" (U.S. Department of Health and Human Services, 2001, p. 49).

Developmental theory underscores the desire of criminologists and other social scientists to better understand how and why individuals come to engage in dysfunctional, deviant and/or violent behaviors across the lifespan. Within a lifecourse and "developmental perspective, there are many interesting parallels between the milestones and behaviors of young children and those of young adolescents, with some important differences" (Wolfe & Mash, 2006, p. 11). Specifically, children and adolescents share the highest rates of deviant, noncompliant, and problem behaviors when compared to other age groups (Mash & Wolfe, 2005). Each of these groups is in tremendous periods of growth on physical, emotional, and biological levels (American Psychiatric Association, 2002) and may have difficulty regulating their emotions. An important difference between younger children and adolescents, however, comes from the amount of self-reliance, responsibility, autonomy, and experimentation with different roles seen in maturing youths. "An understanding of all the different changes taking place during adolescence provides the foundation for understanding the observed rise in risk behaviors and changes in emotional and behavioral problems" (Wolfe & Mash, 2006, p. 11).

As discussed at length previously, however, there is a substantial body of evidence regarding the continuation of problem behaviors over the lifecourse (Blumstein, Cohen, Roth, & Visher, 1986; Sampson & Laub, 1990), as well as the link between early problem behaviors and later aggression (Farrington, 1995). "The stability of behavior is often difficult to gauge prospectively. However, looking back over individuals' lives, it is often more apparent which types of behaviors in an individual's life are stable or not" (Loeber et al., 1998, p. 3). From a developmental perspective, many behaviors are age-appropriate or more likely to occur at certain ages rather than others. Taken within this context for childhood or adolescent behaviors, many acts are appropriate when considering the developmental stage of the person (Popper, Ross, & Jennings, 2000). The question remains whether types of mental health issues may be clinically indicative of maladaptive or pathological problems.

Certainly, a developmental approach, which records the health, histories, and behaviors of subjects over the lifecourse, may offer valuable insight in explaining violent behaviors. Utilization of prospective, longitudinal designs that follow people over the lifespan helps to uncover protective factors that might prevent poor life outcomes and mitigate maladaptive mental health development. The identification of factors that contribute to the prediction of violent behaviors represents one of the main goals of this study.

Aims of the Current Study

Clearly, the levels of violent and chronic offending remain unacceptably high, especially with respect to urban at-risk youths. Such data beckon further inquiries into the possible causes and correlates of violent behaviors and how these predictors may contribute to both the onset and persistence of juvenile types of offending. To date, few studies have focused on the onset of aggression or violence in younger children. Instead, most scholarly inquiries have begun with the critical stage of human development known for impulsive, irrational, and immature behaviors— adolescence. This period signifies a time when "lifelong attitudes, skills, and behaviors are formed as young people respond to family, social, and environmental influences that affect their lives" (Jenson & Howard, 1999, p. 14). The turbulence of adolescence provides a perfect opportunity to challenge one's boundaries. Moreover, the chance to display irrational, immature actions and/or thoughts may lead some youngsters toward pathways of violent and antisocial behaviors. For a small percentage of these youths, this violence trajectory will persist into adulthood.

Recent longitudinal studies have also shown that youngsters in early and middle childhood frequently exhibited multiple problem behaviors across various domains that began at young ages. Some of these youths then progressed into more serious offending later in adolescence or young adulthood (Loeber & Farrington, 2000; 2001). Troubled youths in the criminal justice system have often reported various familial and psychopathological problems that have been linked to delinquency and adult offending (Dembo et al., 1998; Lynam, Caspi, Moffitt, Loeber, & Stouthamer-Loeber, 2007). "It is clear from the literature that young offenders display behavior problems prior to their entry into the juvenile justice system at an early age" (Offord, Lipman, & Daku, 2001, p. 95).

The aims of the current study are to build upon this body of literature and further contribute to the identification of specific mental health factors in childhood and adolescence that may lead to violence and the continuance of serious offending over the lifecourse. This study utilizes a psychosocial approach, relying heavily upon the developmental/lifecourse work of Rolf Loeber and his colleagues at the University of Pittsburgh (e.g., Loeber, 1982; Loeber & Dishion, 1983; Loeber & Le Blanc, 1990; Loeber, Green et al., 1992; Loeber & Hay, 1994; Loeber & Keenan, 1994; Loeber, Russo, Stouthamer-Loeber, & Lahey, 1994; Le Blanc & Loeber, 1998; Loeber, Farrington, Stouthamer-Loeber, & Van Kammen, 1998; Loeber et al., 2005; Fabio et al., 2006; Lynam et al., 2007). This study temporally examines the ability of psychopathological constructs to predict later violent behaviors by using multiple waves of prospective data collected from "at-risk" inner-city boys participating in the Pittsburgh Youth Study.

A number of longitudinal studies have focused on either the development of mental disorders in children (Kellam,

Ensminger, & Simon, 1980; Angold & Costello, 1993) or on the onset and persistence of antisocial and deviant behaviors in boys (Richman, Stevenson, & Graham, 1982; Campbell & Ewing, 1990; Moffitt, 1990). Few studies, however, have prospectively measured a wide variety of measures regarding the onset of both mental disorders *and* violent behaviors simultaneously (Conduct Problems Prevention Research Group, 2002). The present study contributes to this literature by using multiple informant measures of childhood and adolescent mental health factors to determine their relationship with two types of antisocial behaviors, namely serious theft and violent acts.

This study explores a number of specific questions, including: Do different mental health problems predict different types of delinquency or is the presence of emotional disorders predictive of both theft and violence? Are the outcomes of violence and theft predicted by similar mental health problems or are the youths who commit these deviant acts different from one another? Moreover, are parents and teachers both capable informants of problem behaviors or is one informant a more objective observer than the other at predicting poor outcomes in children and adolescents?

To answer these questions, this study methodologically adopts more continuous forms of mental health disorders rather than purely categorical yes/no diagnoses currently used in psychological and psychiatric practice and within most empirical studies conducted today. Children or adolescents who do not have enough symptoms to reach a strict yes/no clinical diagnosis may still have enough differences, when compared with their "normal" peers, to suggest that their problem behaviors are at a level that suggests special attention and/or interventions. Using innovative scales that allow for a distinction between normal, borderline, and clinical levels of mental health problems, this study examines if select mental health constructs are able to predict theft and violence, respectively at various stages of childhood and adolescence.

Regarding the sample and study design for the Pittsburgh Youth Study (PYS), there are distinct contributions from a methodological standpoint for using these data. When compared to the bulk of research that has studied the etiology of violent behaviors, the PYS has numerous advantages and offers significant methodological contributions.

A review of the literature indicates there are an abundance of studies that have retrospectively investigated violence and homicide. While these types of studies are practical, cheaper, and easier to complete, they have a number of shortcomings. That is, these studies are limited by the potential retrospective memory bias of the participants, are often lacking in comparison groups, and temporally are unable to contribute substantially to our knowledge of childhood contributors to violent behaviors (e.g., Radke-Yarrow, Campbell, & Burton, 1968; see Heide, 1999; 2004 for a discussion). In addition, most studies have focused on adolescent, adult, or referred populations, with only relatively recent designs focusing on earlier childhood (Tremblay, Pagani-Kurtz, Masse, Vitaro & Pihl, 1995).

Few empirical studies have examined children beginning their formal education at or around first grade (e.g., Eron, Huesmann, Dubow, Romanoff, & Yarmel, 1987) and followed them into adulthood. Inasmuch as deviant behaviors have been shown to begin prior to adolescence, research that uses samples of younger children provides the greatest chance to identify mental health problems that influence the development of types of serious offending. By design, the PYS purposefully sampled youngsters, their caretakers, and teachers, beginning in first grade. By doing so, these data allow for temporal investigations and observations regarding the reporting on mental health problems in these youths across a number of domains (e.g., home and school) and from different informants (e.g., parents and teachers).

There are definitive public policy implications that come from such research. Certainly, the review of the literature here points to the critical need to further study salient childhood and adolescent mental health factors that may predict later criminal and antisocial behaviors (Loeber & Farrington, 2001). Indeed, "a prerequisite to targeted intervention programs aimed at preventing offending at a young age is information on the prevalence and distribution of emotional and behavioral problems in the preadolescent age group" (Offord et al., 2001, p. 95).

From a public health perspective, these findings also offer important opportunities to better develop educational and social policies that serve at-risk youths, their families, and their communities. Of particular concern are boys who display "multiple problems," or those violent offenders with co-occurring issues such as mental illness and antisocial behaviors (Loeber & Farrington, 2000; 2001). These boys often have problem behaviors that started early in life, have multiple risk factors that cross domains, and are at greatest risk for becoming chronic, serious offenders. Urban African American youth in particular have been shown to be at increased risk of multiple risk factors that have produced poor child outcomes and tremendous stress for youngsters (Li, Nussbaum, & Richards, 2007).

These public health concerns are embodied in the "concerted efforts by governmental and non-governmental agencies to target the high rates of health-compromising behaviors" (Wolfe & Mash, 2006, p. 5) among youngsters. The dominant philosophy for funding and policy strategies on a national level is to identify and understand various types of behavioral and emotional dysfunction that may bring about negative life outcomes for children and adolescents. Few are more critical from a policy perspective to understand than the etiology of violent and aggressive behaviors in youth.

In summary, this study contributes to the literature on the etiology of violence on numerous levels. By using prospective data, the findings of the present study have the potential of offering valuable insight into whether the development of mental illness may predate other negative outcomes, such as aggressive behaviors at younger ages, which put youngsters on violent lifecourse trajectories. Offord and colleagues (2001) recently argued that "more work needs to be done to improve the predictive accuracy of early symptoms for future difficulties" (p. 115). Although there are certainly limitations regarding what the present findings may dictate toward public policy, this work represents another step toward better understanding what childhood and adolescent mental health problems may be related to violence and other types of serious offending.

CHAPTER 2

Exploring the Relationship between Childhood Mental Health Problems and Violent Behaviors

In the United States, mental health problems have come to the forefront of the public consciousness through large-scale public information campaigns, medical shows and reality television, grassroots mental health movements, and more formal education on the specifics of various conditions that afflict children and adults (Flynn, 1987; Wahl, 1995; Phelan & Link, 1998). Mental health problems are defined herein as psychiatric diagnoses, borderline or clinical levels of scores on mental health rating scales that indicate a degree of psychological dysfunction. These scoring instruments come from the work of Achenbach and colleagues, which will be further introduced in detail in Chapter 3. For the purposes of discussion within this paper, the terms mental health problems, mental illnesses and disorders, and psychopathological issues are used interchangeably and refer to this same basic concept of clinical mental health dysfunction.

"Many longitudinal studies have now confirmed that children identified during preschool or early grade school as having severe problems with anger, aggressive behavior, and overactivity tend to continue problematic behaviors in elementary school, adolescence, and young adulthood" (Popper et al., 2000). These investigations of the early onset for violent behaviors over the past 80 or so years have largely come from within the field of psychology.

19

More recently, the major disciplines of anthropology, sociology, public health, epidemiology, and criminology have integrated with psychiatric and psychological disciplines to create a more global perspective on the genesis of violence (Andrews & Bonta, 2003). A large body of scientific evidence has subsequently emerged under the umbrella of lifecourse criminology to study the onset, persistence, and desistence of a wide range of psychosocial problems and deviant behaviors under a developmental framework (see Farrington, 2005, for a review).

When considering issues of critical concern in our schools and communities, the development of serious mental health issues in childhood, their damaging consequences, and how to treat them, is a prominent topic for parents, educators, policymakers, and social scientists (U.S. Department of Justice, 1995). Besides the social costs of violence and other poor life outcomes that appear to be related to the onset of mental health dysfunction, there are also significant long-term economic costs that can be traced to these problems (Wolfe & Mash, 2006). However, "aggression and related behaviors in the young are complex, heterogeneous conditions with diverse etiologies and consequences" (Connor, 2002, p. 2). Due to the salience of these issues, the onset and persistence of select childhood or adolescent mental health problems across various developmental stages, as well as the possible influence of these mental health issues on subsequent violent behaviors later in the lifecourse, is the dominant social problem addressed here. In particular, this study focuses on the ability of four specific childhood or adolescence types of psychopathology in predicting violence, including: Oppositional Defiant, Attention Deficit/Hyperactivity, Anxiety, and Affective Disorders.

Estimates range on the proportion of Americans that believe mental illness leads to violence, with one study reporting that a full quarter of adults endorse this viewpoint

(Monahan, 1992). Another survey found that 36 percent of Americans believed that the mentally ill were more prone to violence, 45 percent believed it was natural to be afraid of these persons, and 52 percent believed in the recognition of former mental patients as potentially dangerous (Link & Steuve, 1994). Obviously, these studies highlight the perception by many people that mental disorders and violence are invariably related and that psychiatric disorders make individuals more prone to aggressive behaviors without warning or provocation (Nunnally, 1961; Link, Cullen, Struening, Shrout, & Dohrenwend, 1989; Link, Phelan, Bresnahan, Steuve, & Pescosolido, 1999). Yet the danger that the majority of individuals who have mental illness pose to others is actually quite minimal (Swanson, Holzer, Ganju, & Jono, 1990; Monahan, 1992; Marzuk, 1996; Angermeyer, Cooper, & Link, 1998). A recent U.S. Surgeon General report on mental health found, "after weighing the evidence…that the contribution of mental disorders to overall violence in the US…is very small" (U.S. Department of Health and Human Services, 2001, p. 49).

The Mental Illness-Violence Link

To be clear, it should be stated that violence in and of itself is not a mental illness; the presence of a mental disorder does not ensure that someone will become violent. While an abundance of research has come forward to support these statements, the same literature suggests that some types of mental illness do play a role in the development of violence, or vice versa (Mulvey, 1994; Connor & Steingard, 1996; Mullen, 1997; Loeber, Green, Lahey, & Kalb, 2000; Swanson et al., 1990). To truly understand this relationship, "we should also be aware of sequences between different mental disorders that may be relevant for the understanding of the development of delinquency and violence" (Loeber, 2004, pp. 40). From a public health perspective, the "clinical recognition of an underlying psychiatric disorder in the aggressive child is important for specific treatment interventions that may diminish aggression as an associated symptom of the psychiatric diagnosis" (Connor, 2002, p. 57).

Concerns about the comorbidity between poor mental health and violence are found throughout the literature. "When we compare the results from population studies with studies in patients with psychiatric institutions and with delinquents in juvenile detention or institutions, the proportion of juveniles with psychiatric disorders is substantially larger" (Loeber, 2004, p. 39). Within the juvenile justice system, an increasing number of youths with mental health problems are entering and remaining within the system, with few effective intervention strategies to treat these offenders (Cohen et al., 1990; Dembo, Cervenka, Hunter, & Wang, 1999; Wasserman, Miller, & Cothern, 2000).

In a recent assessment by Cocozza and colleagues (2005) of a Miami-Dade Juvenile Assessment Center diversion program, the authors renewed the call for comprehensive mental health and substance-abuse assessment and referral services for justice-involved youths and their families. Historically, juvenile offenders have been largely underserved with regard to their mental health needs, despite increasing numbers of these youths being assigned a dual diagnosis for substance abuse and comorbid psychiatric disorders (Dembo, Williams, Wish, & Schmeidler, 1990; Dembo, Turner, Borden, Schmeidler, & Manning, 1995). Overall, studies have shown that juveniles in the criminal justice system have higher rates of mental disorder than their non-delinquent peers (Otto, Greenstein, Johnson, & Friedman, 1992; Andrews & Bonta, 2003). Within one large metropolitan detention center, for example, 20 percent of youths had affective disorders, 23 percent had anxiety disorders, 44 percent had substance abuse problems or disruptive disorders, and at least 80 percent of all youngsters were diagnosed with at least one form of serious psychopathology (Loeber &

Farrington, 2001). A recent synthesis of numerous studies regarding the rates of disorders in mentally disordered juvenile offenders found that between 10 and 88 percent had mood disorders, between two and 76 percent had attention-deficit hyperactivity problems, and 46 and 88 percent of these youths had some form of substance dependency or usage (Boesky, 2002). Scores of other children who have been severely traumatized due to violence exposure or abuse can be found in the welfare, child protective and family court systems; the majority of these children will not receive adequate services for their mental disorders (Harris, Lieberman, & Marans, 2007).

While the onset for mental health problems may start in childhood or adolescence (Patel et al., 2007), these issues continue to have long-term consequences that greatly afflict adult incarcerated populations as well. A recent study by Blaauw and colleagues (2000) reported that between 62 percent and 89 percent of adult prisoners had at least one or more psychiatric illnesses during their lifetime. The early identification of mental illness in youngsters is an important goal for researchers who are trying to determine if a causal relationship exists between various forms of mental disorder and offending. One recent study found only partial support for the criminalization hypothesis, with oppositional defiant problems increasing the risk of arrest, attention deficit/hyperactivity problems having no effect, and internalizing problems such as anxiety and affective issues lowering the risk of criminal arrest (Hirschfield, Maschi, White, Traub, & Loeber, 2006). Others argue that a "not insignificant amount of aggressive behavior occurring in institutions such as psychiatric treatment facilities and in the community may be associated with an underlying psychiatric condition that may or may not be recognized at the time the aggressive behavior occurs" (Connor, 2002, p. 63).

Although some psychiatric disorders are first diagnosed in childhood and have a marked and sequential progression into other disorders in adulthood (e.g., Oppositional Defiant

Disorder), others lack age-specificity (e.g., Affective Disorders) per recognized psychiatric classification systems (American Psychiatric Association, 2000). While the empirical literature shows a somewhat inconsistent association between mental disorders and violent behaviors depending on the disorder, gender, or the population studied, there does appear to be stronger relationships between particular disorders and criminal behavior than others (Bartol & Bartol, 2005). One influential community-based project, the Epidemiological Catchment Area Study, found that subjects were significantly more likely to be violent as the number of psychiatric disorders rose, with risk levels varying from two percent for those persons with no diagnoses to 22.4 percent for individuals with three or more disorders (Swanson et al., 1990).

A review of the body of literature exploring the role of mental health disorders and later violence shows that, for both longitudinal and cross-sectional studies, many of these works have utilized adults, case studies, clinical, and/or incarcerated populations (Cocozza, Melick & Steadman, 1978; Taylor et al., 1994; Gendreau, Little & Goggin, 1996; Bonta, Law, & Hanson, 1998; Hanson & Bussiere, 1998; Heide, 1999; Mullen, Burgess, Wallace, Palmer, & Ruschena, 2000; Curran & Renzetti, 2001; Andrews & Bonta, 2003). Certainly before the 1970s, the majority of research on the relationship between mental health and violence was based on early works of individual studies, retrospective designs, and anecdotal evidence. "Much of the earlier work, therefore, was imperfect, because it was based on highly biased samples, unreliable criteria for judging mental disorder, difficulty in distinguishing case and effect, use of imperfect and incomplete file research, and reliance on official records of delinquency rather than the comprehensive self-reports" (Loeber, 2004, p. 15).

These studies, while a meaningful step toward understanding the complex relationship of mental illnesses with types of antisocial behaviors, are obviously quite limited in their generalizability and methodologies. To address these limitations, the present study attempts to make a substantive contribution to the literature by using prospective, longitudinal data that followed inner-city boys who participated in the Pittsburgh Youth Study. In some measure, each of the psychopathological disorders included here has been recognized as significantly affecting youngsters' outcomes and has been posited as a valid predictor of future violence. This study design and methodology allows for consideration of the temporal order of how mental illness and violence may co-exist.

While the specific design and methods used here to explore this topic will be discussed in substantial detail in the following chapter (Research Design & Methods), the discussion now turns toward explaining the official categorical classification system regarding psychopathological disorders. Next, the reader is familiarized with four mental health disorders that have been empirically linked to violence and which are of interest here. Again, these mental health issues include Oppositional Defiant, Attention Deficit/Hyperactivity, Anxiety, and Affective Disorders. The relevant definitions, criteria, and prevalence of each disorder are provided. In addition, these disorders are discussed briefly as they may relate with other poor developmental outcomes over the lifespan, including violence.

Classification of Mental Disorders

The clear need to develop an official nomenclature for mental disorders led the American Psychiatric Association (APA) to develop the first manual of mental disorders in 1952, or the Diagnostic and Statistical Manual: Mental Disorders (DSM-I) (American Psychiatric Association, 2000). The revised fourth text version, or the DSM-IV-TR, was published in 2000 and is the current guide for clinicians, academics, and practitioners across a wide range of disciplines. This publication allows for the definition and diagnosis of over 400 mental disorders and is the dominant classification manual in the U.S. (Comer, 2004).

A lengthy history of the significant transformations that have occurred within the DSM is beyond the scope of the current study. Briefly, the text has mirrored similar changes in theoretical direction that have been seen in psychiatry and psychology in general. That is, whereas the first and second versions of the DSM were deeply influenced by Freudian theory and psychoanalytic thought, the later editions have moved away from subjective, causal, and theoretical foci. Instead, the third edition "tried to eliminate theory and etiology and concentrate on description and classification, although it is debatable to what extent that was accomplished" (Bartol & Bartol, 2005, p. 191). In the fourth edition of the DSM-IV-TR, "behavioral patterns and psychological characteristics...are clustered into diagnostic categories" (Andrews & Bonta, 2003, p. 358). These categories are based largely on empirical and clinical evidence, with considerable effort made toward a consensus regarding criteria, mechanisms, prevalence, and sequences of disorders when applicable. Five axes are used to record information on individuals, with the first two of these classification axes focusing specifically on mental disorders (American Psychiatric Association, 2000).

Within the DSM-IV-TR, "each of the mental disorders is conceptualized as a clinically significant behavioral or psychological syndrome or pattern that occurs in an individual and that is associated with present distress (e.g., a painful symptom) or disability (i.e., impairment in one or more important areas of functioning) or with a significantly increased risk of suffering death, pain disability, or an important loss of freedom" (American Psychiatric Association, 2000, p. xxxi). There must be a negative consequence for the person from the existence of the mental condition. Thus, a certain number of criteria must be present *and* these criteria must also be "considered a manifestation of a behavioral, psychological, or biological dysfunction in the individual" (American Psychiatric Association, 2000, p. xxxi). This categorical system further states that the behaviors, thoughts, and motivations of individuals diagnosed with mental disorders cannot be a product of expected coping mechanisms or normal functioning. There must be some type of dysfunction present within the person's internal processing system. However, "at present there is no unified, overarching theory of aggression in psychiatric disorders that allows for a single classification system to explain all the variegated presentations of aggressive behavior" (Connor, 2002, p. 63).

Critical Perspectives on Categorical Nature of DSM

A large body of literature has been produced across psychology and psychiatry that criticizes the categorical nature of the DSM (Spitzer, Williams, & Skodol, 1980; Frances, Pincus, Widiger, Davis, & First, 1990). In response to these critiques, dimensional, non-categorical approaches to studying mental illness have also risen in prominence in the field. "These approaches often result in a dimensional approach to aggressive and antisocial behaviors in which symptoms are continuously distributed in a population, without a clear 'cutoff' that identifies them as being present or absent" (Connor, 2002, p. 111). Intense debate continues as to whether distinct boundaries can be made using categorical classifications to distinguish between normative versus psychopathological behaviors (Klein, Lewinsohn, & Seeley, 1996; Regier et al., 1998). "A more realistic goal might be to develop arbitrary but reasonable and meaningful quantitative points of demarcation along more continuous distributions of functioning" (Widiger & Clark, 2000, p. 950).

Critics of mental disorder classifications have also argued that since the "diagnostic process depends to a considerable degree upon clinical judgment, it is easy to label almost all serious offenders as having a mental disorder" (Andrews & Bonta, 2003, p. 358). Others have argued that the race of the clinician or clients may influence clinical diagnoses of mental health disorders (Pottick, Hsieh, Kirk, & Tian, 2007). To minimize such indiscriminate classifications, a good number of objective and standardized instruments have been developed. For example, tests such as the Child Behavioral Checklist (CBCL) are frequently used and have been widely accepted as valid and reliable (Robins & Helzer, 1994; Millon, 1996; Loeber et al., 1998; Andrews & Bonta, 2003). In addition, these types of standardized instruments have been converted to capture information from multiple informants (e.g., parents and teachers) as a way to provide a more holistic picture of problem behaviors across distinct domains (e.g., home and school). With regard to mental health problems in children, for instance, "the importance of multiple informants for an adolescent's emotional/behavioral problems has been well accepted in developmental research on psychopathology" (Phares & Danforth, 1994, p. 721). The use of multiple informants is an important methodological decision and strengthens the design of this body of work.

"Certain mental disorders of childhood have been linked to the later development of violence. They may be early indicators that a child is at increased risk of becoming an aggressive or violent adult; or the disorder may promote later violence by making a child harder to socialize and by evoking negative responses from family, peer, and teachers" (Meadows & Kuehnel, 2005, p. 190). It should be noted, however, that while the DSM-IV-TR stipulates that ODD and ADHD are generally disorders typically first diagnosed in childhood or adolescence, they can also be clinically identified later in the lifespan as well. The onset of psychiatric disorders in childhood is a serious public health and social concern for academics, clinicians, and families alike.

In a recent executive summary report by the National Institute of Mental Health (2001), a committee of experts reported that "childhood neuropsychiatric disorders will rise by over 50% internationally to become one of the five most common causes of morbidity, mortality, and disability among children" (p. 1). Although most children are unruly, disruptive, or recalcitrant at various times in their growth cycle over the lifespan, such behaviors become problematic when they *regularly* interfere with their functioning, sometimes across a number of domains. Indeed, psychiatrically impaired children typically exhibit impairments across several domains simultaneously, including family, school, and peers (U.S. Department of Justice, 1995; Heide, 1999). In an effort to better understand those disorders in childhood or adolescence that may be linked empirically to violence, the following section examines relevant definitions, criteria, prevalence, and empirical associations with violent behaviors for several serious psychopathological problems investigated here.

Mental Disorders with Common Onset in Childhood and Adolescence

Oppositional Defiant Disorder

ODD is diagnosed as a "recurrent pattern of negativistic, defiant, disobedient, and hostile behavior toward authority figures that persists for at least six months and is characterized by the frequent occurrence of at least four of the following behaviors: losing temper, arguing with adults, actively defying or refusing to comply with the request of rules of adults, deliberately doing things that will annoy other people, blaming others for his or her own mistakes or misbehavior, being touchy or easily annoyed by others, being angry and resentful, or being spiteful or vindictive" (American Psychiatric Association, 2000, p. 100). The DSM notes that the "symptoms of the disorder are typically more evident in interactions with adults or peers whom the individual knows well, and thus may not be apparent during clinical examination" (American Psychiatric Association, 2000, p. 100). Moreover, when compared to their peers, ODD children display these symptoms at much greater frequencies and to the point that their academic and social functioning is negatively impacted.

While some people have an initial onset of ODD in adolescence, many others who display ODD symptoms as youngsters will outgrow these behaviors in their adolescent years (Boesky, 2002). The typical presentation of ODD symptoms, however, is in preschool or early childhood (McMahon & Forehand, 2003), with a select group of these disturbed youths continuing across the lifespan to develop the more serious disorders of Conduct Disorder (CD) in later childhood or adolescence and Antisocial Personality Disorder (APD) in adulthood (see Routh, 1994; Lahey, Miller, Gordon & Riley, 1999; Verhulst et al., 2001; National Institute of Mental Health, 2001). Studies have strongly argued that ODD is a precursor to adult deviance (Langbehn et al., 1998). If youths meet the necessary CD criteria for diagnosis, then CD supersedes an ODD diagnosis. CD is recognized as "a repetitive and persistent pattern of behavior in which the basic rights of others or major age-appropriate social norms or rules are violated" (American Psychiatric Association, 2000, p. 98). Although some of the CD criteria involve law-breaking behaviors, other symptoms are not based on illegal acts.

ODD is recognized as one of the early "disruptive behavioral disorders" (Boesky, 2002) that appears to be significantly related to poor life outcomes over the lifecourse, including violence (Farrington, 2005). ODD disruptive behaviors are less severe than CD and "typically do not include aggression toward people or animals, destruction of property, or a pattern of theft or deceit" (American Psychiatric Association, 2000, p. 101). Other common associated features of ODD include low personal self-image, moodiness, a low frustration threshold, profanity, and comorbidity with substance and alcohol usage (Connor, 2002).

The prevalence of ODD varies greatly throughout the epidemiological and psychosocial literature. The DSM-IV-TR reported prevalence for ODD that ranged from two percent to 16 percent, depending upon the study and sampling designs (American Psychiatric Association, 2000), and these rates are similar to those found in other recent studies (Landy & Peters, 1991; Campbell, 1995). Other researchers have placed rates in the general population between three percent and nine percent (see Anderson, Williams, McGee, & Silva, 1987; Kashani et al., 1987), between two percent and 30 percent of clinically referred preschoolers (Beitchman, Wekerle, & Hood, 1987; Lee, 1987; Sprafkin & Gadow, 1996), and between 80 percent and 91 percent for incarcerated youths (Davis, Bean, Schumacher, & Stringer, 1991).

Prevalence in males has been reported to be considerably higher than in females, especially in pre-pubescence, with gender estimates ranging between six percent to 16 percent versus four percent to nine percent, respectively (Cohen, Cohen, & Brook, 1993; Zoccoulillo, 1993). Some longitudinal community samples have seen lower rates of prevalence in boys, with Loeber and colleagues reporting that 2.2 percent of 7-year-olds, 4.8 percent of 11-year-olds, and 5 percent of 13-year-olds had an ODD diagnosis within the Pittsburgh Youth Study (Loeber et al., 1998). Once disruptive behaviors are present within youths, however, the stability of these problems has been the same or greater in girls as in boys (Tremblay et al., 1992; Loeber, Burke, Lahey, Winters, & Zera, 2000). There is a lack of consistent conclusions with regard to the onset of ODD as a function of age (see Cohen et al., 1993; Lewinsohn, Hops, Robert, Seeley, & Andrews, 1993; Loeber, Burke et al., 2000).

Epidemiological estimates of youngsters meeting an ODD diagnosis ranged across study designs and populations, with between 7 percent and 26 percent of youngsters examined meeting criteria across studies (Richman & Graham, 1975; Earls, 1980; Campbell, 1995).

Of particular importance to clinicians is that these types of disruptive youths make up between one-third to one-half of clinical referrals. Even more problematic is the fact that the prevalence of disorders such as ODD continues to increase in children and adolescents (Webster-Stratton, 2000, p. 387).

The possible relationships between ODD and aggression have alternately been posited to be more of an indirect one (August, Realmuto, Joyce, & Hektner, 1999). For youths who did progress on from ODD to CD early in the lifecourse, ODD was a significant predictor of poor outcomes later in life (Loeber, Lahey, & Thomas, 1991; Lahey & Loeber, 1994; Lahey et al., 1995), much as previous CD diagnoses in persons with APD have been linked to a poorer prognosis in adulthood (Lahey et al., 1994; August et al., 1999; Loeber, Burke, & Lahey, 2002). A great number of those children who developed ODD never progressed on to a diagnosis of CD, however (American Psychiatric Association, 2000). From this review, the present inquiry into whether ODD may influence offending behaviors at various stages of childhood and adolescence will be a valuable contribution to the body of developmental and lifecourse criminology.

Attention Deficit/Hyperactivity Disorder

Attention Deficit/Hyperactivity Disorder, or ADHD, is another widely recognized childhood disorder. There is frequent comorbidity of this disorder with ODD (Frick, 1998). Some experts consider this disorder to be synonymous with hyperactive syndrome, minimal brain dysfunction, hyperkinesis, and attention deficit disorder (Bartol & Bartol, 2005).

According to the DSM-IV-TR, ADHD is characterized by a persistence of symptoms of at least six months in duration, leading that individual to become dysfunctional in multiple settings (American Psychological Association, 2000). These criteria must be regarded as unacceptable for a person of that developmental and age level. Specifically, individuals must display six or more criterion with regard to 1) inattention (e.g., carelessness/inattention to detail, difficulty paying attention, inability to listen, difficulty organizing, frequent loss of important items, inability or reluctance for sustained mental tasks, failure to complete assignments/tasks, easily distracted, forgetful), and 2) hyperactivity-impulsivity (e.g., often fidgets, leaves assigned seating, running/climbing excessively, difficulty playing quietly, excessive energy, talking excessively, blurting out answers, inability to wait turn, interrupts others' activities or conversations) (American Psychological Association, 2000, p. 92). Obviously, there is a great heterogeneity of behaviors that encompass this disorder, but the symptoms of hyperactivity are typically present before age seven (Waslick & Greenhill, 1997).

As with ODD, there must be a clear indicator that the presence of the disorder has disrupted at least two of the social, academic, or occupational settings for that individual. To diagnose this disorder, criteria must not be more appropriate for diagnoses for schizophrenia, Psychotic Disorder, Pervasive Developmental Disorder, or mood, anxiety, or dissociative disorders (American Psychological Association, 2000). Moreover, symptoms must have been present prior to age seven.

Three distinct subtypes have been identified in ADHD disordered individuals. That is, ADHD diagnoses include: 1) ADHD-predominately inattentive type (ADHD-PI), 2) ADHD-predominately hyperactive/impulsive type (ADHD-PHI), and 3) ADHD, combined type (ADHD-C). ADHD-PI appears to be more associated with poor academic outcomes and information processing (Lahey et al., 1994). In contrast, some research has suggested a sequential progression of preschoolers with ADHD-PHI into ADHD-C as older children (Loeber et al., 1992; Barkley, 1996; 1998).

The prevalence rates for ADHD vary depending upon the age, gender, sampling and study designs, much like for

ODD. Regardless of the reporting source, however, ADHD is now recognized as the leading psychiatric disorder in American children (Bartol & Bartol, 2005). In the U.S. alone, it was reported that approximately eight million males and two million females live with ADHD (Cowley, 1993). ADHD is not purely an American phenomenon, with this diagnosis being reported in every country tested thus far (Connor, 2002). Most estimates of the childhood populations worldwide hover between three percent and five percent overall for this psychiatric disorder (Offord, Boyle, & Racine, 1991; Wolraich, Hannah, Pinnock, Baumgaertel, & Brown, 1996; Rapport & Chung, 2000), with some pediatricians reporting that four percent of their patients have this disorder (Wolraich et al., 1990).

ADHD has been reported to comprise 30-60 percent of clinical referrals in child psychiatry in the U.S. (Rapport & Chung, 2000). Estimates for the disorder ranged from three percent to seven percent in the DSM (American Psychological Association, 2000); other scholars have reported figures from one percent to 20 percent across populations (Szatmari, 1992; Barkley, 1998; Rapport & Chung, 2000). Younger children and males appeared significantly more likely to be diagnosed with ADHD than were adolescents or females, with some researchers estimating boys to outnumber girls by four to one (Ross & Ross, 1982). Males outnumbered females by ratios of 2:1 to 5:1 in some studies (Szatmari, 1992). A troubling observation was that over two-thirds of children diagnosed with ADHD continued to display symptoms well into adolescence (Rapport & Chung, 2000).

Outcomes for Individuals with ADHD

Children with ADHD have difficulties building strong and healthy interpersonal relationships. That is, "as research on ADHD accumulates, it is becoming increasingly apparent that ADHD is not so much a disorder of activity as it is a *disorder of interpersonal relationships.* Even those children who are not aggressive and who manage to control some of their 'hyperactivity' still have problems with their social interactions" (Bartol & Bartol, 2005, p. 65). The fact that so many ADHD youngsters are brash, loud, and offensive to those around them makes it difficult for them to forge friendships, attachments, and positive interactions with their families, teachers, or peers (Henker & Whalen, 1989; Reid, 1993). More relevant to the mental health focus within this paper are concerns regarding "the central problem of disinhibition [of ADHD symptoms in predicting] negative outcomes in adolescence and adulthood, including increased problems with aggression, antisocial behavior, social skills deficits, poorer occupational functioning, and persistence of ADHD symptoms" (Connor, 2002, p. 71).

Children diagnosed with ADHD also reported higher levels of delinquent and deviant behaviors in adolescence and adulthood, especially when these disruptive actions began between the ages of five and seven years old (Moffitt & Silva, 1988). A minority of all ADHD children (at most 20-25%) have been found to go on and exhibit persistent antisocial offending patterns in adulthood (Rapport & Chung, 2000). Those persons that did so developed criminal career trajectories and committed serious acts, including violence (Moffitt, 1990; Satterfield, Swanson, Schell, & Lee, 1994; Broidy et al., 2003). When compared to children without the disorder, youths with ADHD were at significantly greater risk of both delinquent behaviors and disruptive conduct disorders (Hinshaw, Lahey, & Hart, 1993; Angold, Costello, & Erkanli, 1999; Waschbusch, 2002). Indeed, numerous longitudinal studies have found that ADHD children displayed "a higher rate of externalizing behavior disorders and an increased risk for aggressive behavior, delinquency, and other antisocial behaviors" (Connor, 2002, p. 73) when compared to children without this mental disorder.

Based on these past observations, it seems logical that there is great comorbidity between ADHD and types of disruptive disorders (Loeber & Schmaling, 1985; Pliszka, 1998; Voeller, 1998). Researchers have estimated that between 50 percent and 75 percent (Safer & Allen, 1976) of referred children had ADHD-CD in combination with one another. "In part, the elevated rate of comorbid disorders among treated or treatment seeking populations reflects the fact that multiple co-occurring disorders lead to greater psychosocial deficits than a single disorder" (Bauer & Houston, 2004, p. 504). In addition, poor academic outcomes, truancy, and inflated high school failure rates of over 25 percent of these youths have frequently been reported (Rapport & Chung, 2000). Other researchers have found that children with ADHD have more severe, persistent, and aggressive conduct problems than those without this disorder (Abikoff & Klein, 1992).

Anxiety Disorders

Upwards of 19 million Americans are estimated to suffer from various anxiety disorders and these mental problems are among the most common psychiatric illnesses afflicting both adults and children (Anxiety Disorders Association of America, 2006). The course of these types of "internalizing" disorders generally includes early age of onset, chronicity, and relapsing or recurrent illness (Marcus, Olfson, Pincus, Shear, & Zarin, 1997). The DSM-IV-TR (2000) categorizes several forms of anxiety problems that are included in the present study design and which are therefore presented here. These disorders are common in children and adolescents and are argued by some researchers to be a "protective factor for decreasing the expression of aggression" (Connor, 2002, p. 106). Briefly, these disorders include Generalized Anxiety Disorder, Social Phobia, and Specific Phobia.

Generalized anxiety disorder

Generalized Anxiety Disorder is characterized by at least six months of persistent and excessive anxiety (American Psychiatric Association, 2000). This criterion must be accompanied with difficulty in controlling such unrelenting, chronic worry. At least three additional symptoms for adult diagnosis must be present and include: restlessness, being easily fatigued, lack of concentration, irritability, muscle tension, and disturbed sleep. In children, only one of these symptoms must be present (American Psychiatric Association, 2000).

The diagnosis of Generalized Anxiety Disorder is contingent upon the subject not meeting criteria for another form of anxiety disorders (such as Panic Disorder, Social Phobia, Obsessive-Compulsive Disorder, Separation Anxiety Disorder, Posttraumatic Stress Disorder), or having another type of psychiatric condition such as Somatization Disorder, Eating Disorders, or Hypochondriasis. These persons typically have significant impairment in their functioning due to excessive and chronic worry, which negatively impacts their social, occupational, and academic domains. Another important feature of this disorder is that the intensity, duration, and frequency of the anxiety are greatly out of proportion to the likelihood or concern that an event should cause. Children with Generalized Anxiety Disorder tend to focus overly on their performance and competence in their grades, sporting activities, family, health, acts of nature, and being timely for deadlines and goals (Anxiety Disorders Association of America, 2006). Older children tend to endorse more symptoms than youngsters, with one study reporting that worry about future events was the common symptom (Strauss, Lease, Last, & Francis, 1988).

Associated features with Generalized Anxiety Disorder include "trembling, twitching, feeling shaky, and muscle aches and soreness" (American Psychiatric Association, 2000, p. 473). These persons may also complain of numerous physical complaints due to their constant state of anxiety, including insomnia, abdominal upset, and profuse sweating, accelerated heartbeat, shortness of breath, and dizzy spells, but these symptoms may be quite sporadic. Frequent comorbidity with Mood Disorders such as Major Depressive Disorder and Dysthymia Disorder is also common, as is the diagnosis of other Anxiety Disorders such as Panic Disorder, Social and Specific Phobias, and substance abuse problems.

Prevalence estimates for Generalized Anxiety Disorder in community samples ranged from one percent over a one-year period (U.S. Department of Health and Human Services, 1999) to more than five percent over the lifetime and to approximately 25 percent of all referred anxiety patients in clinical settings (American Psychiatric Association, 2000). Girls tended to be more likely than boys to have this disorder by a ration of 2:1 (Brawman-Mintzer & Lydiard, 1996), with 50 percent of all cases having early onset in childhood or adolescence (U.S. Department of Health and Human Services, 1999).

Social phobia and specific phobia (social anxiety disorder).

Social phobia is a persistent fear of situations in which the child is exposed to possible scrutiny by others, and fear that he or she may act in a way that will be humiliating or embarrassing" (Rabian & Silverman, 2000). The DSM-IV-TR further states that exposure to social or performance situations results in immediate anxiety responses in these individuals, and while children may not recognize that their responses are unreasonable, adolescents or adults typically do (American Psychiatric Association, 2000). For people under the age of 18, persistent symptoms of fear, avoidance, and distress must persist for at least six months with peers and not just adults; these symptoms significantly inhibit the routine, occupation, or social life of the person. These negative outcomes have been shown to have serious psychosocial implications for youngsters, especially adolescents (Ialongo, Edelsohn, Werthamer-Larsson, Crockett, & Kellam, 1995).

"In children, crying, tantrums, freezing, clinging or staying close to a familiar person, and inhibited interactions to the point of mutism may be present. Young children may appear excessively timid in unfamiliar social settings, shrinking from contact with others, refuse to participate in group play, typically stay on the periphery of social activities, and attempt to remain close to familiar adults" (American Psychiatric Association, 2000, p. 452). These fears may lead to avoidance behaviors of certain social situations (Ballenger et al., 1998), shyness, and social inadequacy (Kagan, Reznick, & Snidman, 1988). Moreover, these symptoms must be independent of another general medical condition or another psychiatric disorder (such as Panic Disorder, Separation Anxiety Disorder, Body Dysmorphic Disorder, a Pervasive Developmental Disorder, or Schizoid Personality Disorder). Physical complaints due to severe stress over these situations may include heart palpitations, tremors, shaking, quakes, gastric distress, muscle tension, blushing, and confusion (American Psychiatric Association, 2000).

Prevalence rates for Social Phobia in the DSM-IV range across the epidemiological and scholarly literature, with reports from community samples between three percent and 13 percent. Other studies have reported that between 10 percent and 20 percent of all persons diagnosed with anxiety disorders have this disorder (American Psychiatric Association, 2000). A recent U.S. Surgeon General Report put the one-year prevalence rates for Social Phobia at roughly between two and seven percent (U.S. Department of Health and Human Services, 1999).

Specific Phobia has many similar characteristics to Social Phobia, with the essential feature of the disorder described as a "marked and persistent fear of clearly discernible, circumscribed objects or situations" (American Psychiatric Association, 2000, p. 443) such that exposure to the specific feared event or stimulus evokes an instantaneous stressful response. As with Social Phobias, children with Specific Phobia may be unable to recognize that their reaction is unreasonable when compared to adolescent or adult subjects with similar fears. For individuals under 18 years of age, these persons must have the symptoms for at least six months to meet a formal diagnosis. As with other psychiatric disorders discussed here, Specific Phobia symptoms must be severe, persistent, and/or frequent enough to negatively impact the social, occupational, and academic domains of the person. Common sources of fears include spiders, dogs, bees, storms, speaking, snakes, or heights, which can be brought on by an incident or reinforced by family members (U.S. Department of Health and Human Services, 1999). "This inordinate fear can lead to the avoidance of common, everyday situations" (Anxiety Disorders Association of America, 2006, p. 2).

The associated features of Specific Phobias can involve a disturbance of lifestyle or habits to avoid the stimulus or fear, with typical onset in childhood or early adolescence and another peak in the early 20s for other individuals (U.S. Department of Health and Human Services, 1999). This psychiatric disorder is commonly found to co-occur with other types of Anxiety Disorders, Mood Disorders, and Substance-Related Disorders (American Psychiatric Association, 2000). Five common subtypes of Specific Phobia are detailed by the DSM-IV and include 1) Animal Type, 2) Natural Environment Type, 3) Blood-Injection-Injury Type, 4) Situational Type, and 5) Other Type. It is common for children to outgrow fear of animals and acts of nature as they grow older. Females are more than two times more likely than men to have such afflictions. While phobias are certainly common in society, the level of impairment is typically not reached by most conditions to warrant this diagnosis.

Depending upon the threshold used to measure dysfunction and the type of the specific phobia, community samples cite prevalence rates range between four percent and 8.8 percent, lifetime rates between 7.2 percent and 11.3 percent, and childhood prevalence between two and three percent, with significant declines in the population as they age (American Psychiatric Association, 2000). The U.S. Surgeon General recently estimated the rate of Specific Phobia at roughly eight percent of adults nationwide over a one-year period (U.S. Department of Health and Human Services, 1999).

Generalized Anxiety Disorder, Social Phobia, and Specific Phobia clearly have much in common with respect to their onset, course, and prevalence rates. The overall prevalence of various forms of anxiety disorders is argued by some experts to be the highest of all psychiatric conditions commonly occurring in childhood and adolescence (Costello et al., 1996). There is comorbidity with other serious disorders as well, with some studies reporting between 22 percent and 33 percent of children with externalizing problems in community samples also having a form of anxiety disorder (Russo & Beidel, 1994). Unlike ODD and ADHD, however, youths with anxiety disorders typically have been found to be *less* likely to commit violent acts, with some studies positing that anxiety mediates other forms of disruptive problem behaviors, especially in boys (Walker et al., 1991). Most importantly to the present study, anxiety disorders such as these may serve as a potential protective factor against aggressive behaviors, especially when found to co-occur with oppositional behaviors (Connor, 2002). However, the negative social and psychological consequences of anxiety disorder for youngsters afflicted with these disorders is still not completely understood, especially as it may relate to longitudinal studies on certain types of offending behaviors, and warrants further investigation.

Affective Disorders

Mood disorders, or affective disorders, include several different diagnoses within the DSM that have overlapping symptomology. Mood refers to the emotions or feelings that a person experiences daily. For example, healthy individuals are expected to feel happy, sad, elated, disappointed, angry, or tired depending on the situations they face during a day. These emotions, however, are kept in control and within the social contexts of acceptable manners to cope with these emotions.

Two of the most commonly diagnosed disorders afflicting children and adolescents within the affective or mood disorder group are Major Depressive Disorder (MDD) and Dysthymia, and are discussed below. Historically, depressive symptoms in children and adolescents were largely ignored in developmental psychology prior to the 1980s. Due to the influence of the dominant psychological theories at that time, there was great controversy surrounding the "normality" of childhood depression. Consequently, there was a paucity of research until relatively recently, when depressive disorders in the young became recognized as a valid psychiatric condition (Stark, Bronik, Wong, Wells, & Ostrander, 2000).

Individuals with MDD and Dysthymia are largely unable to control their emotions. "Their intense moods often interfere with daily activities, including their ability to interact with others, attend school or hold a job. They often have physical complaints and may withdraw from friends and family" (Boesky, 2002, p. 62). These affective symptoms may lead to other poor life outcomes that can negatively impact individuals over the lifecourse, with a substantial body of literature linking forms of depressive disorders with aggression and violence.

Major depressive disorder

Major depressive disorder, or MDD, has been studied extensively over the past 20 years and has become one of the most commonly diagnosed and recurring psychiatric conditions in children and adolescents (American Academy of Child and Adolescent Psychiatry, 1998). MDD results in feelings of isolation from proximal reference groups (e.g., family, teachers, peers) for those persons diagnosed with this disorder. "Interpersonal and family relationships are often severely impaired during an episode of MDD" (Connor, 2002, p. 76). Depression episodes produce intense periods of emotions characterized by hopelessness, worthlessness, and in extreme cases, suicidal thoughts. Most people are assumed to have a depressive episode at one point in their lives. "It has often been said that depression is the equivalent of the common cold in psycho-pathology...major depression is among the most common reasons for seeking psychiatric help and hospitalization in the general population" (Millon, 1996, p. 287).

The DSM-IV-TR states that the essential feature of MDD is a symptom of extremely depressed mood or loss of interest that lasts for a minimum of two weeks. In addition to these two symptoms (one of which must be present), four more of the following must also be present almost daily: 1) significant weight loss or gain or irregular appetite, 2) insomnia/excessive sleeping, 3) psychomotor agitation or retardation, 4) fatigue or loss of energy, 5) feelings of worthlessness or excessive guilt, 6) inability to concentrate or communicate, and 7) recurrent thoughts of death or suicide (American Psychiatric Association, 2000, p. 356).

In addition, these symptoms must not meet criteria for Mixed Episode, which includes episodes of mania with depression (see DSM for more information), cannot be due to medication prescribed or abused, and cannot be part of a normal bereavement process. It is critical that these symptoms cause impairment across social, occupations, or other vital areas of functioning. Major depressive episodes can be mild, moderate, or severe. MDD may be diagnosed for a single episode or a recurrent status. To be considered recurrent, two or more episodes must be present at least two months apart.

The prevalence of MDD varies according to age and the population studied. Generally, reviews across numerous studies have suggested that rates of MDD were lower in younger children (0.4%-2.5%) when compared to adolescents (0.4%-8.3%), older adolescents (20%-24%) and lifetime prevalence in adults (10%-25% for women and 5%-12% for men) (see Fleming and Offord, 1990; Birmaher et al., 1996; Hammen & Rudolph, 1996; Goldstein, Walton, Cunningham, Trowbridge, & Maio, 2007). One-year prevalence rates for youngsters have been estimated to be under one percent for young children and up to eight percent for teenagers in other studies (Anderson & McGee, 1994; Kessler & Walters, 1998). In a recent review, the U.S. Surgeon General estimated that five percent of children and adolescents between the ages of nine and 17 had major depression (U.S. Department of Health and Human Services, 1999). Thus, from a developmental perspective, it appears that younger children are at less risk of developing MDD than are adolescents.

With respect to gender, studies have found girls and boys in early childhood had an equal likelihood of being diagnosed with MDD (Birmaher et al., 1996). When looking later in the lifecourse, other studies have reported that females were significantly more likely to develop MDD in adolescence than were males (7.6% versus 1.6%, respectively) (see Cohen et al., 1993). Andrews and Bonta (2003) reported prevalence rates across criminal populations of 1.1 percent to 17 percent in a recent meta-analysis across eight studies on mental illness. Importantly, evidence has mounted that persons born in the later part of the 20th century are developing MDD at greater rates than those persons born prior to this time (Kovacs & Gatsonis, 1994; American Psychiatric Association, 2000).

While much research has been conducted on depression in adults, studies on MDD in children were sparse prior to the 1980s. Prior to this time, "debates over the existence of depression in childhood dominated the literature and it is very likely that these debates delayed relevant research" (Stark et al., 2000, p. 291). In the past 25 years since this time, "research has established that MDD in children and adolescents is a valid psychiatric disorder that can be reliably diagnosed by clinicians, is common in youth, and is a recurrent disorder that often runs in families" (Connor, 2002, p. 76).

Criteria are generally the same for children and adults. One notable exception with respect to depressed children in associated features, however, is that motor agitation may be expressed as aggressive behaviors in youngsters (Barlow & Durand, 2002). Indeed, "school officials, parents, law enforcement, and counselors may be diverted by the aggressive and antisocial behavior of adolescents and may fail to look for and treat an underlying depression" (Meadows & Kuehnel, 2005, p. 201). Relationships with depressed children, especially boys, may be filled with feelings of hostility, irritability, and aggression much more so than in those of adults (Puig-Antich et al., 1985; Knox, King, Hanna, Logan, & Ghaziuddin, 2000). Studies have reported that between 80 percent and 87 percent of depressed youngsters displayed irritable traits (Goodyear & Cooper, 1993; Ryan et al., 1987).

Depression in children and adolescents has also been linked to violent behaviors, such as suicide ideation and attempts (Mitchell et al., 1998; Goldstein et al., 2007), delinquency in adolescence (Kovacs, 1996; Teplin, 2001), and homicidal ideation in adulthood (Birmaher et al., 1996). In addition, "compared to depressed adults, youths suffering from depression have been found to have more guilt, lower self-esteem, and more unexplained somatic complaints" (Connor, 2002, p. 76). Depressed persons tend to have impaired interpersonal relationships, be less sensitive to the feeling of others, and may abuse substances, which in turn may reinforce delinquent or antisocial acts (Loeber, 2004). More recent studies regarding the developmental ordering between depression and delinquency in males have tended to support the conviction that delinquency preceded depression (Beyers & Loeber, 2003) rather than vice versa (Puig-Antich et al., 1989), although there is some variance across populations and genders (Loeber, 2004).

MDD has also been linked empirically with disruptive behaviors in clinical populations of youths (Puig-Antich, 1982; Biederman, Mick, Faraone, & Burback, 2001). Another host of studies have suggested that severe depression in childhood or adulthood, combined with poor outcomes, high irritability, aggression, and comorbidity with conduct disorders, put individuals at greater risk of violent behaviors and the development of Antisocial Personality Disorder (APD), intermittent explosive disorder (Olvera, 2002; Haller & Kruk, 2006) and Substance Abuse Disorders (SUDs) in adulthood (Birmaher et al., 1996; Puig-Antich et al., 1989; Kasen et al., 2001). Similarly, high rates of co-occurrence have been reported between MDD and ADHD in youngsters; these children were also at greater risk of violence (Zoccoulillo, 1992; Biederman et al., 2001). Empirical studies have also suggested that MDD puts individuals at increased risk for bipolar disorder if the onset of the depression occurs early in childhood or adolescence (Kovacs, 1996; Connor, 2002). Again, high levels of anger, hostility, and aggression have been reported in youths with these comorbid disorders.

Dysthymia disorder

According to the DSM-IV-TR, the essential features of Dysthymic Disorder (DD) include a chronic, depressive mood throughout most days for a minimum of one year within a two-year period for adults or a one-year period for children or adolescents. Individuals may be symptom free for up to two months at a time and must not meet a diagnosis of MDD. If a subject meets a diagnosis for Dysthymia during the first two years and subsequently has a Major Depressive Episode, the person may be dually diagnosed with MDD and Dysthymia thereafter, also known as double depression. During periods of depression, these persons may be overly self-critical and must report at least two of the following symptoms, including: lack of appetite or binge eating, insomnia or hypersomnia, low energy levels, poor self-esteem, lack of concentration and inability to make decisions, and feelings of despair or hopelessness (American Psychiatric Association, 2000).

This psychiatric disorder may not be diagnosed if the person has had Manic Episode, Mixed Episode, Hypomanic Episode, or Cyclothymic Episode, or if the depressive symptoms occur during a Schizophrenic or Delusional Disorder (see DSM-IV). These symptoms cannot also be part of a disturbance for a physiological or other medical condition and must negatively impair the person in their social, occupational, or academic areas of functioning (American Psychiatric Association, 2000). Another important feature of this disorder is the recognition within the DSM of specifiers, such as early onset (prior to age 21), late onset (age 21 or older), and atypical (such as mood reactivity, which is more common in females).

The associated features of Dysthymic Disorder are quite comparable to MDD, but tend to be fewer and more chronic in their persistence. These symptoms commonly include "feelings of inadequacy; generalized loss of interest or pleasure; social withdrawal; feelings of guilt or brooding about the past; subjective feelings of irritability or excessive anger; and decreased activity, effectiveness, or productivity" (American Psychiatric Association, 2000, p. 378). In contrast to MDD, the duration of Dysthymia is much longer in children, with a typical course of three to four years (Kovacs, Obrosky, Gastonis, & Richards, 1997; Connor, 2002). It is quite common for these youths to consequently develop MDD soon thereafter, especially in those persons who present early in life with this psychiatric condition, with up to 11 percent of Dysthymic children becoming diagnosed with MDD within a year (Stark et al., 2000; Connor, 2002). For youngsters, the DSM-IV reported that Dysthymia was found to frequently co-occur with MDD, disruptive disorders, and ADHD (American Psychiatric Association, 2000; see also Kovacs, Feinberg, Crouse-Novak, Paulauskas, & Finkelstein, 1984; Kovacs, Akiskal, Gatsonis, & Parrone, 1994). Arguably, the most common co-occurring psychiatric condition with depressive disorders overall is Anxiety Disorders, however (Brady & Kendall, 1992).

Both boys and girls appear to have equal rates of prevalence of Dysthymia in childhood, with youngsters presenting as overly cranky, pessimistic, lacking social skills, and poor self-image (Rutter, 1986). Once in adolescence, however, the diagnosis of Dysthymia is twice as common in girls when compared to boys (Linehan, Heard, and & Armstrong, 1993). Prevalence rates for this disorder hovered between three and six percent, with higher percentages for persons with comorbid MDD (American Psychiatric Association, 2000). Other estimates have placed the prevalence of Dysthymic Disorder in adolescents at approximately three percent (Garrison et al., 1997). For MDD and Dysthymia, other studies have placed estimates between two and five percent within the general population (Stark et al., 2000). Additional studies have reported that 70 percent of Dysthymic youths will also have MDD (Kovacs et al., 1984; Kovacs et al., 1994).

Empirical evidence has linked both MDD and Dysthymia in childhood and adolescence to later anger and violence in these subjects (U.S. Department of Health and Human Services, 2000), with some scholars arguing that this relationship with aggression may be mediated due to the suppression of resentment in youths (Blumberg & Izard, 1995). Kashani and colleagues found substantiation that this dysfunctional relationship between aggression, anger, and other depressive symptoms may begin very early in life, with Dysthymic youngsters under the age of six displaying physically aggressive behaviors in a sample of clinically-referred children (Kashani, Dahlmeier, Borduin, Soltys, & Reid, 1995; see also McGee & Williams, 1988). Other studies have produced contradictory findings, with these scholars reporting that a poorer prognostic course of depressive symptoms was more likely when onset occurred after puberty (Harrington, Fudge, Rutter, Pickles, & Hill, 1990).

Conclusions on Mental Health

There are several substantive and public policy reasons to study a variety of mental health disorders, particularly in males, given their disproportionate representation in serious offending (Loeber, Farrington et al., 2003). First, mental health problems can be destructive and debilitating on their own (Patel et al., 2007). These disorders can have significant negative effects on the lives of persons who live with them, as well as society as a whole (Farrington, 2005). Secondly, research indicates that the prevalence of serious disorders with onset in childhood and adolescence, such as ODD, ADHD, Anxiety Disorders, and Affective Disorders, is rising and constitutes a serious public health concern (U.S. Department of Health and Human Services, 1999). The co-occurrence of these mental disorders increases the chances of maladjustment and dysfunction in the lives of people with these illnesses (Loeber & Keenan, 1994).

Thirdly, there is a need to study these disorders using innovative and dimensional measurement techniques that can distinguish between normal, subthreshold, and clinical levels of impairment (Widiger & Clark, 2000; Achenbach & Rescorla, 2001). Lastly, and perhaps most salient to the topic of this paper, each of these disorders have empirically been connected to some degree with violent and aggressive behaviors, yet many of them are still poorly understood (Farrington, Loeber, & Van Kammen, 1990; Connor, 2002; Loeber, Farrington, et al., 2002; Loeber, 2004). As most longitudinal research to date has primarily focused on delinquency and the development of problem behaviors, few of these studies have also looked at other major areas of psychosocial influence (Fergusson, Horwood, & Lynskey, 1994) while temporally controlling for previous problem behaviors.

To date there is a lack of effective and holistic intervention programs "especially needed by minority and inner city youths and their families, who have historically been underserved" (Dembo, Dudell, Livingston, & Schmeidler, 2001, p. 3). Clearly, pioneering mental health programs are greatly needed for such disadvantaged populations in particular (Tolan, Ryan, & Jaffe, 1988; Dembo et al., 1999; Dembo, Schmeidler, et al., 2001; Loeber & Farrington, 1998; Loeber & Farrington, 2000; Loeber, Farrington et al., 2002; Harris et al., 2007). Many times, troubled youngsters' "difficulties can be traced to family alcohol/other drug use, mental health, or crime problems which began at an early age" (Dembo, Seeberger et al., 2000, p. 2). Therefore, by using a developmental perspective of these types of mental illnesses, the present study hopes to make a significant contribution to social science by addressing 1) understanding, 2) treatment, and 3) prevention of serious behavioral problems over the lifecourse.

CHAPTER 3

Developmental Modeling of DSM-Oriented Problems and Serious Offending Behaviors in Youth

Pittsburgh Youth Study Design

As stated previously, the Pittsburgh Youth Study (PYS) is one of the three original OJJDP Causes and Correlates of Delinquency Studies (with sites in Pittsburgh, Rochester, and Denver) that were undertaken in 1987. This prestigious and well-respected study by Rolf Loeber, Magda Stouthamer-Loeber and their colleagues has produced an impressive number of peer-reviewed publications. To date, there are well over 100 articles, two books in print and another in production, and numerous sub-studies published on the PYS boys.

"The key aims of the Pittsburgh Youth Study are to investigate and describe developmental pathways to serious delinquency, the risk and protective factors that influence the development of serious offending, and the prevalence and pattern of help seeking for youth with disruptive and delinquent behavior" (Loeber et al., 2003, p. 94). The study examines substance and mental health problems, school, family, peer factors, and neighborhood influences across a number of informants, including participating youths, parents or caregivers, and teachers (Loeber, Stouthamer-Loeber et al., 2002).

The present study seeks to independently validate the large number of PYS-related publications that have reported a link between DSM-III mental disorders and the development of serious behaviors from a lifecourse perspective.   Despite the large amount of scholarly literature coming from this study, it is unclear how similar PYS boys are with regard to mental health factors when compared to national samples of boys in similar age groups. There is clearly much more to be learned about the temporal relationship between the early onset of mental health problems and what effects they have on negative outcomes later in life, especially with respect to violent behaviors and multiple-problem youths.   This study attempts to contribute toward this understanding by looking at the incidence (rate of onset) across developmental periods and the rates of prevalence (percent of population reporting problems) of various taxonomic forms of psychopathology and then subsequently examining what relationships may exist with self-reported and officially-recorded serious theft and serious violent behaviors as the boys grew out of childhood and adolescence.

Study Methodology

The PYS has longitudinally collected data at regular periods from three cohorts of male inner-city youths who were originally in Grades 1, 4, and 7 when the study was initiated (see Table 1). These three cohorts of youngsters are referred to as the youngest, middle, and oldest samples, respectively.   For screening, approximately 1,100 boys were randomly selected from each of the three grades in the Pittsburgh Public School system and asked to participate in the initial assessment (called Phase S). These youths were assessed in two initial cohorts (one in the spring of 1987 and one in the spring of 1988) and screened for antisocial behaviors. This process resulted in an overall participation rate of 84.7 percent of eligible respondents (Loeber et al., 2003).

From these screenings, the top 30th percentile of the most antisocial youths were identified (or approximately 250 boys in each of the three samples). An additional 30 percent were then randomly selected from the remaining 70

Table 1 *Sequence of Assessments for Youngest, Middle, & Oldest Samples in the Pittsburgh Youth Study.*

C1	1987	1988	1989	1990	1991	1992	1993	1994	1995	1996	1997	1998	1999	2000
C2	1988	1989	1990	1991	1992	1993	1994	1995	1996	1997	1998	1999	2000	2001
	Sp Fa	Sp Fa	Sp Fa	Sp Fa	Sp Fa	Sp Fa	Sp Fa	Sp Fa	Sp Fa	Sp Fa	Sp Fa	Sp Fa	Sp Fa	Sp Fa

Youngest Sample

Age	7	8	9	10	11	12	13	14	15	16	17	18	19	20
Phase	S A	B C	D E	F G	H	J	L	N	P	R	T	V	Y	AA

Middle Sample

Age	10	11	12	13
Phase	S A	B C	D E	F

Oldest Sample

Age	13	14	15	16.5	17.5	18.5	19.5	20.5	21.5	22.5	23.5	24.5	25.5
Phase	S A	B C	D E	G	I	K	M	O	Q	SS	U	W	Z

Note. C1 = Cohort 1   C2 = Cohort 2; Sp = Spring.   Fa = Fall.

percent of boys and also asked to participate, resulting in roughly 500 boys in each of the youngest, middle, and oldest samples (n = 503, 508, and 506, respectively). Thus, half of each final sample was considered high risk and the other half was average or low risk. The combined number of youths participating in the study with all three samples totaled 1,517 males.

The average ages of participants at the screening wave were 6.9, 10.2, and 13.4 years for the youngest, middle, and oldest samples, respectively (see Loeber, Stouthamer-Loeber, & White, 1999). Just over half of the final sample participants were black and just under half were white, which accurately reflected the racial composition of the Pittsburgh school system (race is discussed further in the Control Variables section at the end of this chapter). These participants were initially interviewed at six-month intervals (Phases A through H in Table 1) and then annually thereafter (J through AA in Table 1).

As the present study is concerned with early onset of mental health-related problem behaviors as a predictor for future aggressive behaviors, such as violence, the present study uses data exclusively from the youngest sample, or the participants at the lowest age at entry into the study (see Table 2). For the youngest sample (n = 503), 18 regular assessments have been made (from ages 7 to 20). Over these 18 assessments attrition has been kept to a minimum, with an impressive average participation rate of 82.3 percent being maintained. While approximately 17 percent of the sample has been lost to attrition, analyses have revealed no disproportionate loss for any certain high-risk populations over the course of the study (Stouthamer-Loeber & van Kammen, 1995). When considering both the youngest and oldest samples, these groups "probably constitute the most extensively uninterrupted followed-up sample in the United States, spanning late childhood, adolescence, and early adulthood with information about delinquency, substance use, and mental health problems...[moreover,] there are no gaps in missed

Table 2 *Years and Ages at Assessment for Youngest Sample in the PYS.*

Years	Age of PYS Boys	Phases
1987-1988	7	S & A
1988-1989	8	B & C
1989-1990	9	D & E
1990-1991	10	F & G
1991-1992	11	H
1992-1993	12	J
1993-1994	13	L
1994-1995	14	N
1995-1996	15	P
1996-1997	16	R
1997-1998	17	T
1998-1999	18	V
1999-2000	19	Y
2000-2001	20	AA

assessments in the follow-ups of these samples, which makes it possible to reconstruct the boys' lives in a cumulative manner" (Loeber et al., 2003, p. 97).

What makes the PYS unique is more than just its longitudinal design and regular assessments. The PYS overcomes a number of limitations that have characterized the majority of earlier studies. First, it begins with preadolescent samples in recognition of research that has demonstrated that "an early offset of offending during the elementary school period predicts later chronic offending" (Loeber et al., 2003, p. 93). Secondly, it records baseline measurements of antisocial behaviors, thereby permitting temporal determinations of these behaviors.

Thirdly, its large sample size permits greater generalizability of these findings and allows determinations of causality of those behaviors to be entertained. Fourth, the relatively low attrition rate of this long-term longitudinal study increases the validity of the findings and the statistical power of these data. Finally, "the large and regular number of assessments of subjects made it possible to trace the development of deviancy and the duration of exposure to risk factors, which can only be achieved by regular assessments of risk factors and outcomes at frequent intervals" (Loeber et al., 2003, p. 94). Clearly, through its innovative and disciplined design, the PYS offers improvements to the weaknesses of past longitudinal studies that have previously attempted to explain the causes and correlates of criminal and aberrant behaviors. Furthermore, and most specific to the present study, it offers a unique opportunity to study the temporal onset of childhood mental disorders as a predictor of future problem behaviors, such as oppositional defiant disorder, attention deficit/attention disorder, anxiety disorders, and affective disorders.

To ensure the reliability of these data, Loeber and his colleagues have taken great care with the data collection from the time of initial assessment and throughout the subsequent follow-ups (see Stouthamer-Loeber, 1993; Stouthamer-Loeber & Van Kammen, 1995). Staff members were trained extensively according to a strict protocol and were accompanied in the field on several occasions to ensure reliability. Staff members who made observations while accompanying the interviewers checked interrater reliability. "Further, at each phase, at least 10% of the interviewed families were called by office staff to re-ask some questions that interviewers had missed during the interview and that needed to be retrieved later. Interviewers were aware of the extensive checking procedures, and so far, we have not lost any data because of interviewer incompetence or dishonesty" (Loeber et al., 1998, p. 49). It can be said, then, that the PYS offers a reliable, high-quality, and extraordinarily large amount of longitudinal data that researchers may use to investigate the potential causes and correlates of poor lifespan outcomes.

Nosologically-Driven Approaches to Studying Mental Health

There is a critical need to study how mental health problems may contribute to criminal and antisocial behaviors (Dembo, Wothke et al., 2000; Loeber & Farrington, 2001), especially within the context of how early onset of behaviors may influence serious offending later in life. As such, the identification of mental health factors that contribute to the prediction of theft and violent behaviors is the main goal of this study. Operating under a general mental health framework, optimal mental health is posited here to be related to prosocial lifecourse outcomes. Conversely, the development of mental disorders is expected to be to antisocial outcomes, or specifically serious theft and violent behaviors, over the lifespan.

The current categorical nature of nosologically-driven (or top-down) DSM diagnoses (such as in the DSM-IV-TR) has historically allowed for only dichotomous decisions that state whether enough criteria are present in a person such that a mental disorder is found to be present versus absent (Achenbach, Bernstein, & Dumenci, 2005). This "top down" approach "starts with diagnostic concepts as a basis for categories of disorders...[these] uniform cut-off points for the number of required symptoms, as well as criteria for age of onset and duration, are the same for both genders and different ages" (Achenbach, 2001, pp. 264-265). Thus, the nosologically-based paradigm "works down to the formulation of diagnostic criteria" (Achenbach et al., 2005b, p. 50), which clinicians then use as they gather and assess data through a variety of instruments and methods.

These purely dichotomous and categorical systems of diagnoses within the DSM may preclude youths who have problem behaviors and who do not display enough of the criteria to meet a diagnosis for certain types of child psychopathology. It is well recognized that children are an especially challenging population to diagnose due to issues of variability in normal human development (Hersen & Ammerman, 2000). There is a potential of ignoring or missing important predictor variables about youths who display problem behaviors, by only these DSM-based categorical diagnoses. Moreover, these DSM-based procedures make it "difficult to deal with methodological challenges such as test-retest attenuation and discrepancies among data from different sources, as well as developmental and gender variations in the base rates and clinical significance of symptoms" (Achenbach, 2001, p. 265).

This study joins only a handful to date that have utilized DSM-oriented scales to measure the onset and prevalence of childhood mental disorders in at-risk boys using both multiple informants and multiple waves of data. These DSM-oriented scales were devised by Achenbach and his colleagues (2001) after consulting with 22 cross-cultural mental health experts who determined which descriptive criteria were most consistent with diagnostic categories in the DSM. These symptoms were derived from the American Psychiatric Association's DSM-IV categories of diagnoses for several common child psychiatric disorders, including Oppositional Defiant Problems (ODP), Attention Deficit/Hyperactivity Problems (ADHP), Anxiety Problems, and Affective Problems.

This approach is also considered top-down and nosologically driven, but is based on additive quantitative scores from various gender and age-sensitive instruments and different informants. This technique allows for meaningful comparisons of mental disorders and provides cut-off points, subthreshold scores, and borderline clinical ranges by using DSM-oriented scales of measurement (Achenbach, 2001). These subthreshold ranges allow researchers to identify cases on an individual level that clearly are not "normal," but which do not reach enough criteria to meet DSM diagnoses of mental illness. For the purposes of the present study, these normalized scores allow cohort comparisons on a larger scale to determine what types of mental health problems may temporally contribute to antisocial outcomes, such as violent behaviors. The use of dichotomous, categorical measurement of psychopathology such as DSM diagnoses does not allow for such comparisons. Furthermore, it has been uncertain until now to what extent PYS participants may be similar to and/or different than nationally representative samples of youngsters of similar genders and ages.

This "quantification is especially valuable for personality, genetic, outcome, and longitudinal research in which categorization of disorders as present versus absent may lose important invariations about the severity and purity of particular patterns of problems" (Achenbach et al., 2005b, p. 62). Only a handful of studies to date have utilized this nosologically-driven approach for children or adults (Achenbach & Dumenci, 2001), despite the fact that much of the recent lifecourse literature finds a relationship between early disruptive behaviors and later chronic offending (Farrington, 1986; 1989; Loeber & Dishion, 1983; Loeber & Farrington, 1998; 2000; 2001). There are vital substantive and public policy implications that may come from longitudinal studies of which problem behaviors in young children might predict violent or antisocial tendencies in individuals later in life. Thus, this more continuous form of measurement, while still based on recognized nosological taxonomies, offers a chance to further contribute to our knowledge of how certain mental disorders of childhood may influence serious theft and violent behaviors. In addition, these scales allow for the measurement of comorbid or simultaneous problem behaviors, which is particularly relevant when studying the etiology and correlates of different disorders found in multiproblem youths.

DSM-Oriented Scales

DSM-based profiles display multi-informant data on subjects in relation to the norms for their age and gender (Achenbach & Rescorla, 2001). These DSM-oriented scales are not exact equivalents to a formal DSM diagnosis because they do not include all the specific criteria for all DSM diagnoses. Instead, these scales capture judgments from different informants on a 3-point scale that asks how true a behavior is for a child within two months (teacher-based reports from Teacher Report Form or TRF) or six months (parent-based reports from Child Behavior Checklist or CBCL) of the form being administered. "The associations that are found between diagnoses and scale scores may vary according to the training and orientation of the diagnosticians, the diagnostic procedures, the ages of the children, the sources of data, and other factors" (Achenbach, Dumenci, & Rescorla, 2001, p. 1). In contrast to DSM diagnoses that determine only whether enough criteria are present to meet a specific diagnosis, this "profile indicates how high a child is on each DSM-oriented scale, compared to a national sample of peers of the same age and gender, as rated by the same kinds of respondents" (Achenbach & Rescorla, 2001, p. 45).

These norms are compared to the scores of functioning for other children via a multi-stage national nonreferred probability sampling technique (see Achenbach & Rescorla, 2001, p. pp. 73-80). The normalizing population data were collected in the 1999 National Survey of Children, Youths, and Adults between February 1999 and January 2000 in the 48 contiguous U.S. states. Within randomly selected households, approximately 93 percent (n = 2,029) of parents with children between the ages of six and 18 completed the CBCL; of these respondents, a subsample of youngsters who had not received help for any behavioral, substance abuse, or mental health problems were selected. The scores from this subsample (n = 1,753) were then used to formulate percentiles and T scores for

CBCL profiles falling into a normal, borderline, or clinical range. In addition, different forms of the CBCL were developed to account for possible gender (boys versus girls) and age (6 to 11 versus 12 to 18 year-olds) differences. This ability of DSM-oriented profiles to discriminate based on relevant gender and age differences are a salient point in light of the developmental focus of the present study. For the CBCL sample, 60 percent were non-Latino white, 20 percent were African American, 9 percent were Latino, and 12 percent were mixed or other race.

Similar methods were used to gather information on normative samples of the same children from teachers for the TRF. That is, 72 percent of children who were eligible for school and whose parents agreed to give permission had teachers complete TRF forms ($n = 1,128$). A subsample then created by excluding those students who were previously referred or counseled for a major behavioral or mental health problem in the preceding one-year period ($n = 976$). After determining that no significant differences existed between this 1999 sample and a previous normative sample of youths (1989), Achenbach and his colleagues (2001) combined these groups to form a larger sample ($n = 2,319$) on which calculated percentiles and normalized T scores for DSM-oriented scales for the TRF are based. For the TRF, the national sample had a racial composition of 72 percent white, 14 percent African American, 7 percent Latino, and 7 percent mixed or other race.

For both CBCL and TRF scores, T scores of 50 were assigned to all children who were within the 50th percentile of the normative sample, thereby prohibiting overinterpretations of variance in the differentiation between low scores within normal levels. Such "loss of this differentiation is of little practical importance, because it involves differences that are all at the low end of the normal range" (Achenbach & Rescorla, 2001, p. 89). The borderline clinical range was distinguished by T scores between 65 and 69 (or the 93rd and 97th percentile). Finally, the clinical range was designated by scores greater than 70 (the 98th percentile) and terminating at a maximum score of between 75 and 100, depending on the scale (see (Achenbach & Rescorla, 2001, p. 92).

Using DSM-IV diagnostic categories for emotional and behavioral problems that were particularly relevant for children and adolescents (ages 6 to 18), Achenbach and his colleagues devised a model of six specific problem behaviors, each closely related to a particular DSM disorder or group of disorders. These profiles were based on the ratings of 22 experts in child psychology and psychiatry from 16 cultures around the world. DSM-oriented scales were then created for six discrete types of mental disorder for problem items from the parent (CBCL), teacher (TRF), and youth self-report (YSR) forms that were given a rating of "very consistent" with the associated diagnostic category. These final six DSM-oriented scales included: 1) Oppositional Defiant Problems, 2) Attention Deficit/Hyperactivity Problems, 3) Anxiety Problems, 4) Affective Problems, 5) Conduct Problems, and 6) Somatic Problems.

This study investigated forms of these six DSM-oriented scales: Oppositional Defiant Problems (ODP), Attention Deficit/Hyperactivity Problems (ADHP), Anxiety Problems, and Affective Problems were retained for the analysis. The data for these DSM-oriented profiles were collected on both the parent (CBCL) and teacher (TRF) instruments.

Due to similarities across criteria and scores of young children (Achenbach, Dumenci, & Rescorla, 2000), the Anxiety and Affective Problems pulled items from similar disorders. Specifically, the profile for Anxiety Problems combined like criteria from Generalized Anxiety, Social Anxiety Disorder, and Specific Phobia Disorder. In the same way, the profile for Affective Problems included items from both Major Depressive Episode and Dysthymia.

For methodological and theoretical reasons, the decision was made here not to include two of the problem constructs—or Conduct Disorder (CD) and Somatic

Problems-- in the present study. CD is defined as "a repetitive and persistent pattern of behavior in which the basic rights of others or major age-appropriate social norms or rules are violated" (American Psychiatric Association, 2000, p. 98). While a good number of studies point to the validity of a CD diagnosis (Loeber, 1991; Foley, Carlton, & Howell, 1996; Frick & Loney, 1999), other critics have raised tautological issues within the empirical literature regarding the use of delinquent measures included in a CD diagnosis to predict later criminal behaviors (Millon, 1996). While some of the CD criterion involves legal violations (e.g., using weapons to cause serious physical harm, stealing while victim present), other actions are not serious illegal behaviors necessarily (e.g., stays out a night despite parental prohibitions, uses deceit to obtain goods or services). Although a number of studies have found separate and significant relationships between CD and delinquency (Fergusson & Horwood, 1995; Loeber, Stouthamer-Loeber, & Green, 1991; Burke, Loeber, Mutchka, & Lahey, 2002), CD was excluded in the present analysis to respond to potential confounding issues. The lack of theoretical justification to include Somatic Problems as a possible predictor of future violence rendered it inappropriate for consideration within the confines of this study.

Child Behavior Checklist (CBCL) and Teacher Report Form (TRF) Instruments

To create profiles for the four DSM-oriented scales of concern herein, both parents and teachers gave information on PYS boys that was used to provide systematic comparisons of the same youths across specific domains and multiple data collections. Using parallel versions of the widely used and respected CBCL and the TRF (Edelbrock & Achenbach, 1984), respondents were asked over 120 different items to determine to what extent certain behaviors, attitudes, or feelings occurred within children six months prior to each administration. Responses were coded on a Likert-type scale ranging from 0 to 2 (not true, somewhat or sometimes true, very true or often true). Of these items, 96 behaviors were common across both instruments. In addition, another 10 items were unique to the CBCL and 23 items were specific to the TRF (see Achenbach, Dumenci, & Rescorla, 2001, for more information). These questions related to the mood, behavior, attitude, performance, and the mental and physical health of the boys. Previously published analyses have revealed that correlations between cross-informants were within reasonable levels for reliability and validity (Achenbach & Edelbrock, 1983), with a modest correlation of .28 in a meta-analysis across reports (Achenbach, McConaughy, & Howell, 1987).

These findings indicate that no single source of observation is best; different informants report children in various states of functioning depending upon the context and situation (Achenbach, 2005b). With respect to lifecourse research such as that being conducted here, Achenbach and Rescorla (2001) argue, "data from all available informants can be combined in regression analyses and structural models to optimize associations between ratings and underlying variables that may be etiologically important" (p. 181). Therefore, the use of multiple informants offers a more comprehensive picture of assessment of functioning across domains and situations than a sole informant can provide (Krol, Bruyn, Coolen, & van Aarle, 2006). To get a clear picture of how these domains and data between informants may vary, the present study does not combine measures taken from parents and teachers, but rather keeps them distinct from one another to allow for such comparisons. Indeed, Achenbach et al. (1987) have suggested that it is "essential to preserve the contributions of different informants, even if their reports are not correlated highly" (Renk & Phares, 2004, p. 240; see also Achenbach, 2006; Rescorla et al., 2007).

It should be noted that the 1991 forms of the CBCL and TRF were revised in 2001 in order to create the profiles for the DSM-oriented scales. Previous analyses revealed that the 2001 scales were strongly correlated with similar measures in the syndromes measured on the 1991 forms (r = .74 to .96) (Achenbach & Rescorla, 2001). A few new items were added to accommodate the new scales. Data collected on pre-2001 forms were converted into profiles by omitting a limited number of new items. Of the profiles being considered here, these exclusions from the CBCL were shown to reduce scores only slightly on the Affective Problems and ADH Problems scales; the TRF had reduced scores for DSM-oriented Affective Problems profiles when items were omitted (see Achenbach & Rescorla, 2001). Achenbach and his colleagues did not find that the exclusion of these new items was sufficiently significant as to require special considerations for these DSM-oriented scales.

Data Reduction Strategy

In keeping with other PYS data reduction techniques, the constructs used within the present study were conceptualized with the idea of being "meaningful to lay people as well as professionals so that the results of the analyses could be communicated clearly" (Loeber et al., 1998, p. 49). As such, constructs were created by carefully combining data from the informants across the waves of data collection to make the new DSM-oriented scales. Recall that the "main function of the T scores is to facilitate comparison of the degree of deviance children show across different scales of the same form" (Achenbach & Rescorla, 2001, p. 175). Admittedly, using raw scores allows for all the differences between scores to be analyzed; such analyses, however, make interpretation and comparisons between samples and studies significantly more complex and difficult to interpret.

Achenbach and colleagues do caution in using these *T* scores to do statistical analyses, however, due to the truncation of scores of a minimum of 50 on the low side and a maximum of 100 on the high side. Yet Achenbach and his colleagues also state, "creative research blends ideas, challenges, opportunities, methods, and findings in innovative ways" (Achenbach & Rescorla, 2001, p. 175). While keeping the limitations of such censored (or truncated) data in mind, the present study will use these DSM-oriented scales to contribute to the scientific literature by comparing PYS boys to national samples. As such, this work attempts to better examine how these forms of mental disorder may predict poor outcomes throughout childhood and into late adolescence using a developmental framework.

First, a construct for each phase of data collection was calculated by the primary author, under the direction of PYS staff, using an algorithm that was replicated across all waves of data collection, with the algorithm modified at Phase R for TRF measures (with no reports for Anxiety and Affective Problems) and at Phase T (with no teacher reports available for this phase). Cronbach's alpha (1951) was calculated across each phase of data collection for both parent and teacher reports to measure the internal consistency of each newly formed construct and was found to be within acceptable levels across the phases (see Appendix A). For raw score calculations in each phase, all constructs missing more than 30 percent of the total number of items for each DSM-oriented profile were considered missing. Where fewer than 30 percent of items were missing, values for the missing items were imputed. "Imputation involves filling in values for cases that lack data on a variable based on values of that variable or related variables for cases with valid data" (Miller, 2005, p. 285).

Raw scores were then truncated and transformed in each phase into corresponding *T* scores. These scores were age- and gender- appropriate. That is, for each phase of data collected, the algorithm assigned one set of values for PYS boys ages six through 11 and another for ages 12 through 18. Based upon the specific age of each participant at that phase, an age- and gender-appropriate T score was assigned for that informant. Each T score for the "profile indicates how high a child is on each DSM-oriented scale, compared to a national sample of peers of the same age and gender, as rated by the same kinds of respondent. By contrast, the criteria for the yes versus no DSM diagnosis are the same for children of both genders, different ages, and all sources of data" (Achenbach & Rescorla, 2001, p. 45). After these individual scores were created, they were then "chunked" or blocked together to form developmental age periods to ease in the interpretation of the findings and allow for comparisons with normative samples. When at least one phase of data within an age block was collected for a respondent, values for these missing phases were imputed. For example, if two of the three waves within an age block had data collected, the missing values were approximated by PYS staff for the missing values by using imputation techniques.

Such analyses with normative national samples have never been possible in PYS youths to this point, thus making it difficult to determine to what extent PYS boys are similar to and/or different from other boys within their age groups on a national level. "By being based on percentiles for the normative samples, the T scores provide convenient ways to quickly judge whether parents, youths, and teachers reports higher levels of problems than are reported for nonreferred children" (Achenbach & Rescorla, 2001, p. 176). From the outset, it was expected that due to the oversampling of "antisocial" youths in the PYS, the T scores of these boys would reflect higher means of problem behaviors when compared to national samples that were not oversampled. Despite these expectations, such comparisons have not been possible to date. Accordingly, this study offers valuable insight into how PYS boys of similar ages and genders compare to their national counterparts. Toward this end, Table 3 includes a complete listing of all the time age blocks, corresponding ages of respondents, developmental periods, and instruments used across the age blocks for parents, teachers, and youths for the variables included herein.

Independent Variables: DSM-Oriented Problem Behavior Constructs

Using DSM-oriented scales, then, profiles of PYS boys in the youngest sample were transformed to better understand both the onset of mental disorders in childhood and adolescence and the temporal relationship of how these types of behavioral malfeasance may subsequently influence poor lifecourse outcomes. Prospective, longitudinal data from 14 waves of interviews were collected from parents and teachers residing in inner city Pittsburgh (see Table 2). Borrowing conceptually from the developmental and child psychology literature, these data were "chunked" or "blocked" together to form three age periods that reflect stages of human development during childhood and adolescence.

As shown in Table 3, these stages include Age Block 1 or middle childhood (for the three years between ages 7 through 9), Age Block 2 or late childhood (between ages 10 through 12), and Age Block 3 or early adolescence (ages 13 through 16). That is, Age Block 1 included data collections from Phases A through F (or six bi-annual assessments), Age Block 2 included data from Phases G through L (or two bi-annual and two annual assessments), and Chuck 3 included Phases N through T (or four annual assessments). Both CBCL and TRF instruments were used by the primary author to independently create new constructs for the 4 DSM-oriented scales during PYS Phases A through T (see Appendices B, C, and D for a complete list of the CBLC and TRF items, raw score indices, T-score conversion ranges, and summary descriptive statistics of each mental health problem profile discussed here).

Table 3 *Age Blocked Data Groupings for Independent and Dependent Variables.*

Time Period	Approx Ages	Developmental Period	PYS Phases	Sources/ Instruments
Age Block 1†	7-9 years old	middle childhood	A, B, C,D, E, F	P/CBCL* T/TRF* Y/SRA**
Age Block 2	10-12 years old	late childhood	G, H, J, L	P/CBCL* T/TRF* Y/SRD**
Age Block 3	13-16 years old	early adolescence	N, P, R, T	P/CBCL* T/TRF* Y/SRD**
Age Block 4 ‡	17-19 years old	late adolescence	V, Y, AA	Y/SRD**

Note. Sources/Instruments: Y= Youths/ Self-Reported Antisocial Behavior Scale (SRA) for Phases A-F, and Self-Reported Delinquency Scale (SRD) for Phases G-AA.
† Age block 1 includes data on both the DSM-oriented scales (independent variables) and on physical aggression self-reported by youths (control variable). Age blocks 2 and 3 have data collected for both the DSM-oriented scales and for serious theft and violence behaviors (dependent variables).
‡ Age block 4 includes data for only the dependent variable constructs serious theft and violence behaviors.
* Sources/Instruments: P= Parents/Child Behavior Checklist (CBCL) and T= Teachers/Teacher Report Form (TRF). At Age block 3, for the TRF data were collected for the DSM profiles through Phase P; at Phase R only ODP and ADHP behaviors were collected; at Phase T there are no teacher reports for any DSM-oriented profiles.
** Various instruments were used that were age appropriate for boys throughout the four age blocks of time included here.

Table 4 presents the descriptive statistics for each of the 4 DSM-oriented constructs, including the means and standard deviations for both the PYS and the national normative samples for the CBCL and TRF across the three age blocks. With regard to Oppositional Defiant Problems (ODP), raw scores from five items on the CBCL and TRF were combined to create raw scores for boys ages six through 11 and then for ages 12 to 18. These ODP items on the CBCL included measures such as "argues," "disobedient at home," and "disobedient at school." For the TRF, items were similar but excluded the "disobedient at home" measure and instead offered an item for "defiant" in the school setting. For ODP and all other DSM-oriented constructs, missing data were recoded to a value of 0. If respondents were not interviewed for any phase included in the age block, that subject was coded as system missing for the purposes of analysis (see Table 4 for a total number of these subjects for all DSM-oriented constructs).

Both the CBCL and TRF recorded raw scores ranging from a low score of 0 to a high score of 10 for ODP, regardless of age. These raw scores were then converted into T scores ranging from a low of 50 to a high score of 80 on the CBCL and from 50 to 75on the TRF. As stated previously, normal T scores were rated as those ranging between 50 and 65; borderline scores were those greater than 65 and less than 70; clinical ranges included those boys with T scores of 70 or greater. Neither the CBLC nor TRF had any missing items in converting data from 1991 to 2001 instrument formats for OPD.

As shown in Table 4, the means for ODP for PYS youths across Age Blocks 1, 2, and 3 for the CBCL were 56.64 ($SD = 5.28$), 56.40 ($SD = 5.66$), and 55.90 ($SD = 5.62$), respectively. For the TRF, they were 57.51 ($SD = 6.32$), 58.94 ($SD = 6.86$), and 58.56 ($SD = 6.92$), respectively. These parent reported means were all noticeably higher than those means found in national samples of nonreferred youths, with CBCL national means across similar Age Blocks at times 1, 2, and 3 being reported at 54.80 ($SD = 5.40$), 54.75 ($SD = 5.60$), and 54.70 ($SD = 5.80$). (Please note that the differences between PYS and national means were not statistical difference of means

Table 4 Descriptive Statistics for DSM-Oriented Constructs: PYS and National Normative Nonreferred Samples Mean T Scores and Standard Deviations across Informants and Age Blocks.

	ODD Prob		ADHD Prob		Anxiety Prob		Affective Prob	
	P*	T**	P*	T**	P*	T**	P*	T**
Age Block 1: Ages 7-9								
PYS mean	56.64	57.51	54.85	57.18	53.36	54.49	54.12	55.31
SD	5.28	6.32	4.99	6.11	4.16	4.45	4.29	4.18
n	502	502	502	502	502	502	502	502
Miss-ing	1	1	1	1	1	1	1	1
Nat'l Mean	54.80	53.90	54.10	54.10	54.00	53.80	54.10	53.90
SD	5.40	5.80	5.70	5.90	5.40	5.60	5.60	5.80
Age Block 2: Ages 10-12 †								
PYS mean	56.40	58.94	54.45	58.46	52.82	55.04	52.82	56.13
SD	5.66	6.86	5.24	7.05	3.86	4.93	3.72	4.67
n	483	485	483	484	483	483	483	483
Miss-ing	18	18	18	18	18	18	18	18
Nat'l Mean	54.75	53.85	54.45	54.15	54.20	53.50	54.00	53.90
SD	5.60	5.85	5.60	5.85	5.50	5.55	5.65	5.75
Age Block 3: Ages 13-16								
PYS mean	55.90	58.56	54.01	58.60	52.92	54.71	53.02	55.75
SD	5.63	6.92	4.94	6.96	4.08	5.61	3.95	5.23
n	471	463	471	463	471	458	471	459

Continued on next page

Table 4 continued

Missing	30	40	30	40	30	43	30	43
Nat'l Mean	54.70	53.80	54.20	54.20	54.30	53.20	53.90	53.90
SD	5.80	5.90	5.50	5.80	5.60	5.50	5.70	5.70

Note. The DSM-oriented national means are based upon scored provided by Achenbach and colleagues and do not provide raw data for statistical tests between these national scores and PYS youths.

* P = Parent for PYS and National samples, Parents were given CBCL.

** T = Teacher for PYS and National samples, Teachers were given TRF.

† Age Block 2 means for the National Normative Sample were devised by taking the average of the 6-11 year and 12-18 year-old for means and standard deviations across both the CBCL and TRF. See Achenbach & Rescorla, 2001 (Appendix C) for more information.

tests (*T* tests) due to a lack of available data for the national samples.) For the TRF, national sample means were found to be 53.90 (*SD* = 5.80) for Age Block 1, 53.85 (*SD* = 5.85) for Age Block 2, and 53.80 (*SD* = 5.90) for Age Block 3. These figures indicated that, with respect to ODP, PYS boys appeared to have higher reports from parents and teachers of Oppositional Defiant Problems than comparable national samples of youths of the same gender and ages.

Regarding the frequency of Oppositional Defiant Problem behaviors in PYS boys (see Appendix D), univariate analyses indicated that between 92.8 percent and 91.9 percent of parents rated their sons as having little or no ODP issues over the three age blocks, versus between 77.1 percent and 84.3 percent of teachers reporting normal levels in the same boys. In contrast, parents were less likely than teachers over the three age blocks to report borderline or clinical levels of ODP behaviors in PYS youths, with combined scores ranging from 6.2 percent to 10.1 percent for parents versus 15.7 percent to 22.9 percent for teachers, respectively. Given the oversampling of antisocial youths in the PYS and the caretaker bonds between parents and their children, it is not surprising that teachers viewed PYS boys as having more oppositional behaviors than did the parents of these children.

For Attention Deficit/Hyperactivity Problems (ADHP), seven items from the CBCL were used to create a raw score additive index for all ages of boys. These items included measures such as "fails to finish," "can't cooperate," "can't sit still," "talks too much," or is "impulsive," "inattentive," or "loud." For all boys, scores ranged from a low of 0 to a high of 14. Both age groups (6-11 and 12-18 year olds) had corresponding *T* scores ranging from a low of 0 to a high of 80 on the CBCL. For the TRF, 13 items were used to form the construct, including some similar measures with parents and additional items such as "fidgets," "doesn't follow directions," "talks out," or "disturbs others." These 13 items combined to create a raw score range of 0 to 26 points for all boys between ages six and

18. Missing data were handled as described previously. *T*-score conversions yielded a range of 50 to 80, similar to the CBCL. Again, no items were missing in the conversion of pre-2001 forms.

The descriptive statistics (presented in Table 4) revealed that for parent reports, PYS boys were quite similar in parental reports of ADHP across the time age blocks than national samples, with the exception of Age Block 3. That is, the means at Age Block 1 (*M* = 54.85, *SD* = 4.99) and Age Block 2 (*M* = 54.45, *SD* = 5.24) were close to reports of ADHP of nonreferred children at Age Block 1 (*M* = 54.10, *SD* = 5.70) and identical Age Block 2 (*M* = 54.45, *SD* = 5.60). For Age Block 3, however, PYS boys had a lower mean of ADHP between the ages of 13 and 16 (*M* = 54.01, *SD* = 4.94) than other children (*M* = 54.20, *SD* = 5.50), according to CBCL scores.

In contrast, teacher reports for ADHP were all higher than parental reports for PYS youths, with means across the age blocks reported at 57.18 (*SD* = 6.11), 58.46 (*SD* = 7.05), and 58.60 (*SD* = 6.96), respectively. Nonreferred children had lower reported means than these PYS boys, with 54.10 (*SD* = 5.90) at Age Block 1, 54.15 (*SD* = 5.85) at Age Block 2, and 54.20 (*SD* = 5.80) at Age Block 3. For four out of six comparisons, then, PYS boys appeared to have higher reports of Attention Deficit/Hyperactivity Problems than comparably aged youths on the national level. These findings of higher teacher reports of ADHP for PYS boys were not surprising, again, due to the selectivity of antisocial youths in the study. Additionally, educators in today's society are trained to recognize inattentive and hyperactive traits in children and/or may have less tolerance for behaviors causing disruptions in the classroom. It would seem reasonable that parents may have a different viewpoint of whether their children had these problems at all or that their children did not display the same types of behaviors at home that they exhibited when interacting with their peers at school. Parents may therefore be less likely to acknowledge ADHP behaviors due to the negative connotation that many people now give to such disorders.

Again, univariate statistical analyses (see Appendix D) for each age block showed that parent reports were considerably more in the normal range than were teacher reports of the same boys. That is, whereas parents scored PYS boys between 94 percent and 95.5 percent of the time in normal ranges, only 79.7 percent and 85.9 percent of teachers rated the boys in normal ranges from Age Blocks 1 through 3. Similar to ODP, teacher scores for Attention Deficit/Hyperactivity Problems at borderline and clinical levels (ranging from 14.1% to 20.3%) were also reported at approximately two to five times the rates of parental reports (ranging from 4.5% to 6.0%). Thus, it appears that teachers were again more likely to report frequent ADHP behaviors in PYS boys than were the caregivers.

Combining the same 6 items on both the CBCL and TRF instruments created an Anxiety Problem construct. These measures included items such as "dependent," "fearful of things other than school," "fears school," "nervous," or "worries." Raw scores from both informants ranged from 0 to 12; T scores ranged from 50 to 80 for the CBCL and TRF. No items were missing from conversions from 1991 versions of these forms. For parental reports, a review of the descriptive statistics indicated a change in trends of higher rates of forms of psychopathology in PYS boys when compared to other children. For instance, whereas means for nonreferred samples were found at 54.00 ($SD = 5.40$), 54.20 ($SD = 5.50$), and 54.30 ($SD = 5.60$), respectively, PYS boys' parents reported lower levels of Anxiety Problems for Age Block 1 ($M = 53.36$, $SD = 4.16$), Age Block 2 ($M = 52.82$, $SD = 3.86$), and Age Block 3 ($M = 52.92$, $SD = 4.08$).

These data were in direct contrast to teacher reports, which found the opposite: PYS boys had greater levels of Anxiety Problems than boys nationally. That is, PYS boys were higher at Age Blocks 1 ($M = 54.49$, $SD = 4.45$), 2 ($M = 55.04$, $SD = 4.93$), and 3 ($M = 54.71$, $SD = 5.61$) than nonreferred children ($M = 53.80$, $SD = 5.60$; $M = 53.50$, $SD = 5.55$; $M = 53.20$, $SD = 5.50$, respectively). Univariate analyses (see Appendix D) supported these observations and found that parents reported the vast majority of their children within normal ranges of Anxiety Problems, with percentages between 97.0 and 98.3 of these boys rated as normal and between only 1.7 percent and 3.0 percent of sons in a borderline or clinical range for Anxiety Problems. In contrast, between 91.5 percent and 96.2 percent of teachers reported normal scores, whereas 3.8 percent to 8.5 percent of teachers reported borderline or clinical levels of anxious behaviors. These observations suggest that parents were not viewing anxious behaviors in the same light as teachers or perhaps that these different domains gave varying information about anxiety levels that PYS boys displayed.

Lastly, the construct for Affective Problems was created by adding 12 items to create raw scores (ranging from 0 to 26) for parent reports. While 13 items were included on the 2001 CBCL version, only 12 were available; specifically, "enjoys little" was not measured across the PYS phases and, thus, was excluded and counted as missing in the algorithm. Measures used in the analysis included "cries," "harms self," "sleeps less," "sleeps more," "talks about suicide," "lacks energy," or was "sad." Corresponding T scores ranged from a low value of 50 to a high of 100. TRF raw scores ranging from 0 to 20 were created with nine questions combining to create the additive raw score. The same item on enjoyment was missing for teacher reports. The remaining nine items included mostly the same items as parental reports plus a question about attitudes of apathy. Corresponding T scores ranged from a baseline of 50 to a high of 100.

Similar to reports of Anxiety Problems, PYS parent reports of Affective Problems were generally lower than national averages, with means of 54.12 ($SD = 4.29$), 52.82 ($SD = 3.72$), and 53.02 ($SD = 3.95$) for PYS boys compared to 54.10 ($SD = 5.60$), 54.00 ($SD = 5.65$), and 53.90 ($SD =$

5.70) for the national sample across the time age blocks. Parallel to Anxiety Problem averages, however, teacher reports on the TRF also were higher for PYS boys when compared to other boys. Specifically, PYS means were 55.31 (*SD* = 4.18) at Age Block 1 versus 53.90 (*SD* = 5.80) for the national sample, 56.14 (*SD* = 4.67) versus 53.90 (*SD* = 5.75) at Age Block 2, and 55.75 (*SD* = 5.23) versus 53.90 (*SD* = 5.70) at Age Block 3. These results held true when considering univariate summary statistics (see Appendix D), with normal level of Affective Problems reported between 98 percent and 99 percent of the time for parents versus 93.7 percent and 97.6 percent of the cases for teachers. Very few parents reported borderline or clinical levels of Affective Problems for their sons when compared to teachers' reports, with scores across Age Blocks 1, 2, and 3 ranging from one percent to two percent versus 2.4 percent to 6.3 percent, respectively.

A summary view of these descriptive statistics in Table 4 showed that, for parental reports, higher means for PYS boys appeared across the age blocks, with the exception of Anxiety and Affective Problems, which had lower means for PYS boys, when compared to national nonreferred children (see Figure 1). With regard to teacher reports, PYS boys had higher rates of teacher reports on all DSM-oriented constructs when compared to national samples, including Oppositional Defiant, Attention Deficit/Hyperactivity, Anxiety, and Affective Problems (see Figure 2). When looking across the standard deviations for the PYS versus the national sample, the range of DSM-Oriented values within one standard deviation largely models the same trends we report here with the means. Recall that the national sample racial makeup is quite different from the PYS, with the nonreferred probability sample having a significantly higher proportion of whites and lower proportions of minority/ethnic groups. The fact that the PYS has a much higher representation of disadvantaged minority youths may make this sample at greater risk for mental health problems when compared to these nonreferred normative samples. Thus, care should be used when interpreting these higher T scores for the PYS boys based on these racial differences.

These findings might be explained by the oversampling of troubled youth that occurred in the original study design of the PYS or could be a product of regional conditions unique to Pittsburgh. This sampling design has implications for the interpretation of the summary statistics presented in Appendix D, as well, with the selectivity of antisocial youths being an important caveat for interpreting the percentages presented there. While parents seemed much more willing to rate their children within normal levels, PYS teacher reported a greater proportion of these children in borderline and/or clinical levels of problem behaviors for each of the four DSM oriented scales of interest here. Caretaker bonds and/or parental problem behaviors may render parents as less objective observers of psychopathological symptoms. Parental psychopathology may also be an issue within the family constellation that is reinforcing the mental health problems in these youths. In contrast, teachers may be more willing on a conscious or unconscious level of finding their students in abnormal ranges. This finding points to the need to collect data from multiple observers to allow for the comparison of ratings between domains and informants.

Self-Reported Antisocial Behavior Scale (SRA) and Self-Reported Delinquency (SRD) Instruments

For the dependent variables, similar instruments were used to create self-report data from youths as they grew older. PYS youths were also regularly administered a number of instruments that were developmentally appropriate and that captured self-reported problem behaviors in the six months prior to the data collection. To ensure reliability of the responses and to make certain that all respondents comprehended the questions properly regardless of their

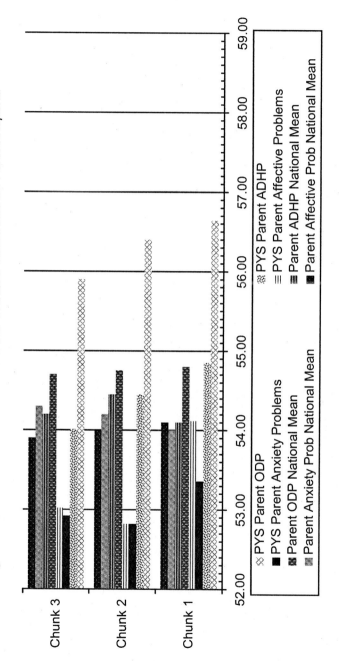

Figure 1. PYS and National Means for DSM-Oriented Constructs for Parent Reports

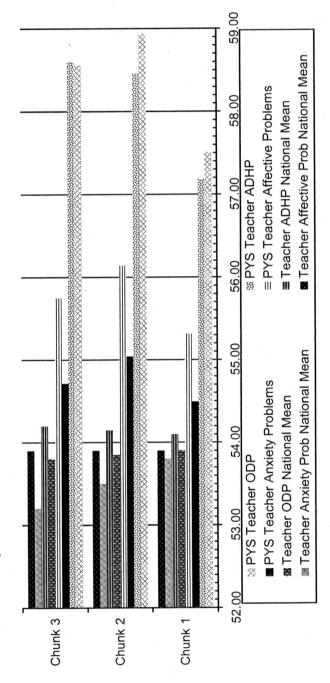

Figure 2. PYS and National Means for DSM-Oriented Constructs for Teacher Reports

Legend:
- PYS Teacher ODP
- PYS Teacher Anxiety Problems
- Teacher ODP National Mean
- Teacher Anxiety Prob National Mean
- PYS Teacher ADHP
- PYS Teacher Affective Problems
- Teacher ADHP National Mean
- Teacher Affective Prob National Mean

literacy level, all items were administered verbally by PYS staff (Loeber et al., 1998).

The first of these questionnaires, given to participating boys in Phases A through F, was the Self-Reported Antisocial Behavior Scale (SRA). To ensure that questions measured behaviors fitting for youngsters, this 33-item instrument sought out reports of lesser measures of delinquency, deceitful behaviors, and substance abuse that were more age appropriate to boys in the first grade. Youngsters were given probing questions and examples by interviewers for more complex behaviors to safeguard against false positive responses (Loeber et al., 1998). Responses were coded as "never," "once or twice," "more often" to accurately capture the prevalence of those behaviors. This instrument was administered to boys in Phases A through F, or the first three years of the study (see Table 2).

The second instrument, given to respondents in Phases G onward, was the Self-Reported Delinquency Scale, or SRD. This 40-item questionnaire was similar to the SRA and was based on the reliable and well-evaluated National Youth Survey (Elliott, Huizinga, & Ageton, 1985). These items pursued information on delinquent acts, lying and deceitful behaviors, theft, and serious violent acts of the youths in the previous six months. These instruments were used to collect self-reported delinquent and criminal behaviors from PYS boys. These reports were then combined by PYS staff with official report data to form the constructs for the dependent variables. Prior to describing these constructs in detail, however, the methodological considerations of using both self-report and official records are explored briefly.

Methodological Considerations Regarding Self-Report and Official Data Sources

There is some controversy as to whether self-reports or official records are the best data sources for studying delinquent and criminal behaviors. Early self-reports were criticized for lacking measures of serious offenses (Hindelang, Hirschi, & Weis, 1976) and the duration and frequency of serious criminal behaviors (Elliott & Ageton, 1980). Some scholars have argued that self- reports may be unreliable measures of delinquent behaviors due to inflated reports for some forms of behavior (Achenbach, Dumenci, & Rescorla, 2002). Conversely, another "proportion of juveniles may not report to an interviewer the extent of their problem behavior, such as the severity of their delinquency" (Loeber et al., 1998, p. 18).

Both the methods and measures of self-reporting have advanced considerably in the past twenty years as more studies have focused on career criminals and lifecourse precursors to serious offending patterns. Indeed, "the development of instruments to better measure serious and very frequent offense and the suggestion to acquire data from high-risk samples coincided with a substantive change in the 1980s in the focus of much criminological work on the etiology of offenders" (Thornberry & Krohn, 2000, p. 40). Self-reports can give valuable information about behaviors and deviant activities that are acted out in a covert manner or that remain undetected by the police (Loeber et al., 1998). Such reports become more valid and reliable when measures include a wide variety of items on delinquency and crime, serious offenses, questions about duration and frequency, and questions that probe these offenses with follow-up (Thornberry & Krohn, 2000).

Regarding official reports, some critics have argued that these data may not accurately portray the true prevalence of some forms of criminal behaviors because obviously not all youngsters are caught for the crimes they commit. Moreover, "objective records may not provide entirely objective evidence…for example, statistics of youth crime may be affected by changing definitions of offense, rate of detection, dispositions by police and courts, and documentation standards" (Achenbach, Dumenci, & Rescorla, 2002, p. 194). For example, only the most serious offenses are included in the Uniform Crime Report, thereby excluding all other less serious crimes committed in the same offense event and diminishing the number of lesser offenses for these situations (Thornberry & Krohn, 2000).

Although official reports have limitations and methodological issues to consider, they are also a rich, available, and extensively used data source. "A more common and more feasible expansion of sources in large studies is to obtain information from official records, such as the records on juvenile offending lodged in juvenile courts or child welfare agencies" (Loeber et al., 1998, p. 19). These official reports can help to reduce the number of false negatives that may come from self-reports (Farrington, Loeber, Stouthamer-Loeber, Van Kammen, & Schmidt, 1996) and provide a larger picture of the criminal activities of respondents than only self-reports allow.

From this viewpoint, there are compelling reasons to combine self-reports and officially reported data to determine the prevalence of delinquent or criminal behaviors within a lifecourse framework (Sampson & Laub, 2001). With respect to the PYS, an analysis by Farrington and colleagues (Farrington et al., 1996) revealed considerable predictive and criterion validity in self-report measures and no significant differences between African American and white males in the likelihood to self-report. These authors also found that approximately two-thirds of boys with court reports admitted such criminal acts on self-reports. These figures are supported by other researchers who have shown similarly strong concordance rates between self-reports and official records, with serious offenses being disclosed less frequently than lesser offenses (Gold, 1970; Elliott & Voss, 1974).

Consequently, for the purposes of this study, the decision was made by Loeber and his colleagues at the PYS to complement self-reports with state and county agency data. These complementary sources "maximize the validity of measurement and strengthen the explanation of delinquency" (Loeber et al, 1998, p. 19) and other types of antisocial behaviors that only a single informant source may fail to report. The self-reports are especially helpful when working with longitudinal data collected more than once annually such as these because it is probable that young children will have very low rates of officially reported crime, but might have self-reports of deviant behaviors that are salient to the purposes of the present inquiry. In addition, due to the complexity of the study design, with the four DSM-oriented constructs, two types of informants, and two dependent variables of interest, to further disaggregate the self-reports from the official data was deemed unnecessary to meet the aims of the research. Thus, both of these data sources were combined to create the dependent variables constructs for both serious theft and serious violence for PYS boys in the youngest sample. Finally, using these specific constructs also was a logical choice because PYS staff had created these variables for other ongoing research and their inclusion here would allow for valuable future cross-study comparisons.

Dependent Variables: Serious Theft and Serious Violence Constructs

Recall that this study is attempting to determine the ability of the DSM-oriented constructs to predict future violent and theft behaviors as PYS youngsters move from late childhood into adolescence. Although the main interest here is concerned with the etiology of violence, serious theft is also included so that distinctions can be made regarding the pathways to particular types of serious offending. With this model in mind, PYS staff created serious theft and serious violence behavior constructs by *chunking* data for the same age periods as those constructed for the independent variables at Age Blocks 1, 2, and 3. However, because this research is concerned with the prevalence of serious criminal behaviors beyond the onset of the DSM-oriented mental health constructs at Age Block

3 (or ages 13 through 16), one further time age block was created for Age Block 4 for the dependent variables. As seen in Table 2, Age Block 4 dependent variable constructs grouped data on serious theft and serious violent behaviors reported in PYS boys when they were approximately 17 to 19 years old. This addition allows for the temporal model to continue through late adolescence, a time known to be critical for adolescents to become involved in deviant, criminogenic, and antisocial acts that may or may not have begun at an earlier developmental period (Moffitt et al., 2001).

With the caveats in mind regarding self-report and official records, the constructs for Serious Theft and Serious Violence were created using each of these data sources. Reports were collected from PYS youths across a number of instruments described previously, including the SRA and SRD. These data were combined with official reports of delinquent behaviors researched in Allegheny County and collected in an Official Records Project (ORP) conducted by PYS staff. These official records were coded by offense date, offense category, and disposition of the offense according to the Federal Bureau of Investigation's Uniform Crime Reports (UCR).

To make the pooled constructs for Serious Theft and Serious Violence, two constructs were first created for the self-reported data collected at each phase. The Theft Self-Report construct included behaviors such as breaking-and-entering and motor vehicle theft. Data were taken from both the SRA and SRD and from parent reports on the CBCL at Phases A through T. The Violence Self-Report construct included forcible theft, attacking a person with the intent to injure, sexual coercion, and forcible rape. Data were taken from the SRD from Phase G onward. The phase constructs were used to make Theft Self-Report and Violence Self-Report for each age block. Age block constructs were assigned a positive score if any phase within the age block was positive and were coded missing if all phases in the age block were missing.

Two parallel constructs were created using the ORP data. Serious Theft Convictions indicated whether the youth was convicted of burglary or auto theft. Burglary is defined here as the entering of a building with the intent to commit a crime (breaking-and-entering). Serious Violence Convictions indicated whether the youth was convicted of robbery, aggravated assault, aggravated indecent assault, homicide, forcible rape, involuntary deviant sexual intercourse, or spousal sexual assault. These data were organized according to the youth's age at the time of conviction. The chunked constructs were then created by determining each youth's age during the phases in the age block and coding the construct as positive if he was convicted at any of those ages.

From these individual self-report and officially reported Theft and Violence constructs, the PYS staff then created a combined construct. The Serious Theft construct combined the Theft Self-Report and Serious Theft Convictions constructs for Age Blocks 1, 2, 3, and 4. The Serious Violence construct was also formed in a similar manner, with the Violence Self-Report and Serious Violence Convictions constructs for Age Blocks 2, 3, and 4. Due to the fact that serious violence information was not available from the SRA and CBCL, no construct could be made for serious violent behaviors in youngsters at Age Block 1, or ages seven to nine. In order to control for other forms of violent behaviors in PYS boys at Age Block 1, a control variable construct called Physical Aggression was created, which will be further discussed in the section that follows.

Table 5 presents descriptive statistics for both of these dichotomous Serious Theft and Serious Violence constructs. This table includes the prevalence of active offending, standard deviations, and sample sizes for Age Blocks 2, 3, and 4 (also see Appendix D for a master summary list of all descriptive variables in the study). As shown here, a small number of youths within the sample were actively committing serious theft behaviors across the age blocks, with 8.0 percent, 16.4 percent, and 6.6 percent of PYS boys, respectively, participating in these behaviors across late childhood, early adolescence, and late adolescence. Similarly, only 10.1 percent, 20.8 percent, and 8.4 percent of respondents, respectively, either self-reported or were formally processed in the criminal justice system for committing violent acts across the three age blocks.

These low rates of offending suggested that, from a developmental perspective, PYS youngsters started to commit both theft and violence at low rates between the ages of 10 and 12 in late childhood, more than doubled these deviant behaviors in early adolescence between the ages of 13 and 16, and then desisted at rates below late childhood as they traveled into late adolescence at ages 17 through 19 years old. These findings were not surprising and are consistent with the age-crime curve reported throughout the criminological and sociological literature whereby a small number of youths display seriously criminogenic behaviors at younger ages, much more do so as adolescents, and the majority of these youths desist from such behaviors as they enter into late adolescence and emerging adulthood (Farrington, 1989; 1995; Elliott, 1994; Moffitt et al, 2001; Loeber & Farrington, 1998; 2000; 2001).

Control Variables: Physical Aggression, Family SES, and Race

Previous research has indicated that several variables are significantly related to longitudinal studies of criminal behavior and, thus, should be included in the analysis. These variables included prior aggressive behaviors (at Age Block 1), family socioeconomic status (for Age Blocks 1, 2, and 3), and the race of the participant. As stated

Table 5 *Dichotomous Dependent Variables: Serious Theft and Serious Violence: Prevalence, Standard Deviations, and Sample Sizes Across Age Blocks.*

	Serious Theft	*Serious Violence*
Age Block 2:		
% Yes	8.0	10.1
% No	92.0	89.9
SD	.27	.30
N	485	485
Age Block 3:		
% Yes	16.4	20.8
% No	83.6	79.2
SD	.37	.41
N	475	477
Age Block 4:		
% Yes	6.6	8.4
% No	93.4	91.6
SD	.37	.28
N	452	453

previously, no data were available on the SRA and CBCL regarding serious violent behaviors for PYS youths at ages seven to nine. Yet previous acts of violent behavior have been shown to influence subsequent reports of violence. Therefore, in order to control for aggressive behaviors at Age Block 1, a construct called Physical Aggression was created from SRA measures and data collections at Phases A through F.

This construct used self-report data from boys in the youngest sample. Measures used in this construct included asking youths to report if they had hit their 1) parents, 2) teachers, or other adults, 3) friends or classmates, and/or 4) siblings in the past six months. Possible scores ranged from 0 to 4 for this scale. The means were calculated for the phases and age block, and then dummy coded for the purposes of analysis (1 = more aggressive and 0 = less aggressive). This dichotomy thereby rated boys as more or less aggressive when compared to the other participants in the sample, with approximately the upper 25th percentile being separated from the lower 75th percentile of boys (see Table 6 and Appendix D for a table of all univariate statistics in the study). These relatively high rates of aggressive behavior at such young ages may be a result of the high prevalence of boys who act aggressively and hit others in late childhood (Loeber et al., 1998). These lesser offenses are more likely to be reported than the serious forms of theft or violent behaviors that are the focus of this study as the boys continued on throughout adolescence.

Family Socioeconomic Status, or Family SES, measured the socioeconomic status of the boys' families. Data provided from the primary caretaker on the Demographic Questionnaire throughout the phases were converted into scores using the Hollingshead (1975) index of social status. This Hollingshead index measure transformed the scale values for occupational prestige into averages across Age Block 1 (42.28) and Age Block 2 (42.30), with a slightly higher mean for Age Block 3 (44.33) on a range of 6 to 66.

These means are remarkably similar across the age blocks, with the slightly higher average for Family SES at Age Block 3 possibly due to increased levels of caretaker educational attainment, higher values of occupational classifications, or job promotions that would be expected over time.

For the purposes of analysis, these age blocked raw scores were subsequently recoded into a trichotomized variable. The values for Age Blocks 1, 2, and 3 of Family SES approximated the top and bottom quartiles and separated these groups from those families in the middle (1= high, 2 = typical, and 3 = low). That is, when

Table 6 *Means, Standard Deviations, Percentages, and Sample Sizes for Control Variables across Age Blocks.*

		Physical Aggression*	Family SES	Race**
AGE BLOCK 1	M	.26	1.98	1.58
	SD	.44	.68	.49
	%	Less aggressive = 75% More aggressive = 25%	Low = 22% Typical = 54% High = 24%	Black = 58% White = 42%
	n	502	502	503
	Missing	1	1	0
AGE BLOCK 2	M		1.98	
	SD		.70	
	%		Low = 22% Typical = 54% High = 24%	
	n		485	
	Missing		18	
AGE BLOCK 3	M		2.01	
	SD		.70	
	%		Low = 24% Typical = 52% High = 24%	
	n		474	
	Missing		29	

Note. SES = socioeconomic status.

* Physical Aggression was only constructed for Age Block 1.

** Race was a constant measured at Screening Phase.

compared to other families within the sample for that age block, the top 25 percent of families with the highest Family SES scores (1 = high) were separated from families with the lowest 25 percent of scores (3 = low), thereby leaving about 50 percent of families classified with typical Family SES (2 = typical). The resulting trichotomous variable was roughly equivalent to a 25/50/25 trichotomy (1 = high, 2 = typical, 3 = upper) because the final percentages were determined by the frequency distributions of the raw scores. These percentages and descriptive statistics for the Family SES variable are presented in Table 6 (also see Appendix D for a table of summary statistics for the variables).

Lastly, a race construct was created from data collected in the Demographic Questionnaire administered to caregivers at the Screening Phase. This construct was recoded and dichotomized (coded 1 = white and 2 = black). In keeping with previous work done by Loeber and colleagues, whites were defined as persons of European or Asian ancestry; blacks were broadly defined as persons of African, Hispanic, American Indian, or mixed ancestry. This race construct has been used extensively in previous PYS studies and the decision to use here will allow for future comparisons across these studies. Descriptive statistics revealed that 58 percent of PYS boys were black and 42 percent were white across the 503 boys in the sample. These percentages were representative of the numbers of black and white children in Pittsburgh public schools and in the original screening cohorts (Loeber et al., 1998).

Methods of Analysis

Due to the categorical and dichotomous nature of the dependent variables, logistic regression was selected as the primary method of analysis, as opposed to OLS regression techniques, for the present study. "The basic concepts fundamental to multiple regression analysis—namely that several variables are regressed onto another variable using one of several selection processes—are the same for logistic regression analysis, although the meaning of the resultant regression equation is considerably different" (Mertler & Vannatta, 2005, p. 313). Moreover, there are key assumptions of OLS regression that are violated by the dichotomous nature of the outcome variables used in the present study. Of particular concern here, multiple regression models assume that 1) there is a linear relationship between the independent and dependent variables in the model, 2) the data are continuous and measured at the interval or ratio level, and 3) the error terms are independent, normally distributed, and have constant variance across the independent variables (Bachman & Paternoster, 2004).

While OLS regression equations use the sums of the weighted and actual values of the predictor variables in order to estimate the values on the outcome variable, logistic regression equations are based on probabilities, odds, and log-odds. Unlike multiple regressions, which assume linear relationships between the independent and dependent variables, logistic regressions model curvilinear relationships and are considerably more flexible than OLS regression models.

A logistic regression equation with k independent variables (X_k) is shown:

$$\text{logit}(p) = \beta_0 + \beta_1 X_1 + \beta_2 X_2 + \ldots + \beta_k X_k + \epsilon,$$

such that p is the probability of the dependent variable with a value between 0 and 1 (Miller, 2005). "Probabilities are simply the number of outcomes of a specific type expressed as a proportion of the total number of possible outcomes" (Mertler & Vannatta, 2005, p. 317). While linear probability models assume continuous values that may fall below 0 and above 1 for the independent variables, probabilities are limited to a range of 0 to 1. The assumptions of multiple regression models are clearly violated with binary dependent variables because the distributions and standard deviations produce curvilinear responses (Agresti & Finlay, 1997).

Whereas probabilities may not be greater than a value of 1, odds may be significantly larger than 1. Odds are defined as a chance of an event happening and divided by the chance of an event not happening, as expressed by:

$$Odds = \frac{p(X_1)}{1 - p(X_1)}$$

where $p(X_1)$ is the probability of the event occurring and $1 - p(X_1)$ is the probability of an event not occurring (Mertler & Vannatta, 2005). These odds are translated into odds ratios (OR) in logistic regression models (Exp(B)), which help to interpret the relative difference between the category of interest and the reference category. If odds are the same of an event occurring between respective and reference categories, then the OR is 1.0. Values above 1.0 reflect higher odds that the event will occur and values under 1.0 mean that there is a protective effect that the event is less likely to occur.

Logistic regression is ultimately based upon the logit or log-odds, which are defined as the natural logarithm of the odds (Mertler & Vannatta, 2005) such that:

$$\ln(p/1 - p) = \beta_0 + \beta_1 X_1 + \beta_2 X_2 + \ldots + \beta_k X_k + \epsilon.$$

Thus, "the estimated coefficient (β_0) from a logistic regression is the change in the natural logarithm of the odds ratio of the outcome associated with a one-unit increase in the independent variable (X_k)" (Miller, 2005, p. 222). Generally, odds ratios are easier to interpret and are therefore used in the results presentation to follow.

Before proceeding with a logistic regression method of analysis, issues regarding potential outliers and multicollinearity were first considered. An examination of the descriptive statistics for the independent variables showed that there were significant issues with skewness and kurtosis due to the transformations of the DSM-oriented construct raw scores to T scores. That is, because these data were censored on the left (at a baseline of 50) and on the right (with a maximum score of 100), the large number of boys who scored within average ranges resulted in a positively skewed distribution for these predictor variables. Thus, the censored nature of the normalized DSM-oriented constructs guaranteed there were no outliers.

However, as this study proposes using binary logistic regression to explore the ability of various types of mental health problems across time to predict future theft and violent behaviors, the potential problem of multicollinearity was of particular concern here. Multicollinearity is an issue for regression analyses because high correlations between independent variables may be indicative that variables are not uniquely contributing to explaining the variance within the model and are thereby violating a key assumption of regression analysis. This violation may result in limitations in explaining the model variance, a confounding of independent variable effects, and an increase in the variance of regression coefficients (Stevens, 1992). To ensure that the independent variables were not highly intercorrelated, a series of tests were performed.

First, preliminary OLS multiple regressions were conducted on the full model so that these correlations could be examined (see Appendix E). This analysis revealed that some of the correlations were greater than .60, suggesting possible temporal correlations for a number of the variables between age blocks. (For example, Attention Deficit/Hyperactivity Problems at Age Block 1 were significantly correlated with Attention Deficit/Hyperactivity Problems at Age Block 2 at a level of .778.) This finding would be an expected one due to the fact that the same problem behaviors are being followed in the same individuals over time. This correlation matrix is admittedly quite complex; although alternative means could have been used to present these data, these analyses would also require both within and between age block comparisons that would be equally cumbersome.

Moreover, while looking at these correlations may be the simplest method to detect multicollinearity, other statistical methods are preferable (see Mertler & Vannatta, 2005). Due to the higher correlations found between some of the variables, these tests included examinations of collinearity diagnostics with respect to either tolerance (Stevens, 1992) and variance inflation factors (VIF) (Norusis, 1998). Tolerance scores range from 0 to 1, with scores lower than .10 indicating high collinearity. High VIF factors, or those variables with a value of greater than 10, also point toward a strong linear association between variables in the model (Mertler & Vannatta, 2005). Perusal of these diagnostics showed that all scores were in acceptable ranges for both tolerance and VIF when held to these recognized standards. Even when using a much stricter rule of VIF > 4, only 23 of 88 possible values were greater than 4.0, with the highest score reported at a relatively modest value of 6.70 for teacher observations of Oppositional Defiant Problems at Age Block 2. Thus, there did not appear to be problematic levels of collinearity between the independent variables.

With respect to logistic regression outputs, there are several principle areas that are typically presented, including statistics for the overall goodness of fit of the model, how accurately the observed values compare to the probability of the predicted values, and the regression coefficients, Psuedo R^2, odds ratios (OR), and predicted probabilities of the variables. To determine the relative ability of the DSM-oriented problems to explain Serious Theft and Serious Violence behaviors above and beyond the control variables, these analyses were conducted in forward blocks and introduced the DSM constructs only in the final step of the model.

Conceptually, there were six models per informant (parent and teacher) and for each type of outcome (Serious Theft and Serious Violence), resulting in a 6 x 2 x 2 design.

As shown in Figure 3, there were six basic temporal models across all the age blocks as follows:

> Model 1: Age Block 2 Dependent Variable regressed on the Age Block 1 Independent Variables.
> Model 2: Age Block 3 Dependent Variable regressed on the Age Block 1 Independent Variables.
> Model 3: Age Block 4 Dependent Variable regressed on the Age Block 1 Independent Variables.
> Model 4: Age Block 3 Dependent Variable regressed on the Age Block 2 Independent Variables.
> Model 5: Age Block 4 Dependent Variable regressed on the Age Block 2 Independent Variables.
> Model 6: Age Block 4 Dependent Variable regressed on the Age Block 3 Independent Variables.

A replication of these six basic models times the two types of respondents equals 12 models; these 12 models are then multiplied by the two types of outcomes, theft and violence, for a total combination of 24 models. The models and the findings from the logistic regression analyses show the long-term prediction ability of parent and teacher reports of DSM-oriented problem behaviors on both Serious Theft and Serious Violence in PYS boys. These 24 distinct models and their findings are presented and discussed at length in the results section.

Figure 3. Example of Temporal Models for DSM-Oriented Constructs in Predicting Theft or Violence across Age Blocks.

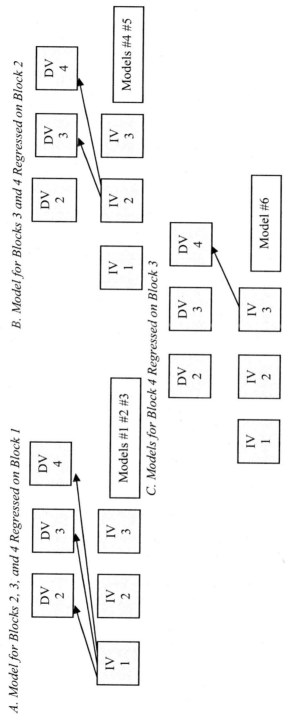

A. Model for Blocks 2, 3, and 4 Regressed on Block 1

B. Model for Blocks 3 and 4 Regressed on Block 2

C. Models for Block 4 Regressed on Block 3

Note. DV = Dependent variable constructs (Serious Theft or Violence Behaviors). IV = Independent variable DSM-oriented constructs for both informants, including parents and teachers. Numbers listed next to DVs or IVs correspond to the time age block for these constructs (e.g., IV 1 = IV at Block 1). Each arrow indicates a separate model, with three models for A, 2 models for B, and 1 model for C.

CHAPTER 4

Findings Regarding Youth Violence and Property Crime

Logistic Regression Models and Subgroups

To date, few studies have utilized longitudinal, prospective data from a developmental perspective to determine the influence of psychopathological behaviors on offending. Toward a better understanding of the contribution of how mental health problems explain such antisocial outcomes, the present study conducted forward block logistic regressions on 24 separate models, each of which examined the long-term predictive ability of DSM-oriented profiles of Oppositional Defiant, Attention Deficit/Hyperactivity, Anxiety, and Affective Problems.

These 24 models test the efficacy of these DSM diagnostic profiles in predicting both Serious Theft and Serious Violent offending by 503 boys in the youngest sample of the Pittsburgh Youth Study. As discussed in the methods chapter (see Figure 3), these 24 models formed a 6 x 2 x 2 design. That is, six basic models were replicated across the age blocks for each respondent (parents and teachers) and for each offense type (Serious Theft and Serious Violence) to form the basic six models.

Thus, the analytic plan resulted in six basic temporally-ordered models tested across two dependent variables and with data provided by two separate sources, producing: six models on the effect of parent reports of DSM problems on Serious Theft, six models on the effect of teacher reports of DSM problems on Serious Theft, six models on the effect of parent reports of DSM problems on Serious Violence, and six models on the effect of teacher reports on Serious Violence. This resulted in a total of 24 logistic regression models, or 12 models per informant (parents versus teachers) and 12 models per dependent variable (Serious Theft versus Serious Violence).

Appendixes F through Q present the results for these 24 logistic regression models in their totality. To ease in interpretation of such a large number of logistic regression models, the tables are laid out for the reader one subgroup at a time, beginning with the effects of parent reports of DSM problem on Serious Thefts later in childhood and adolescence. The subsequent relationships between teacher reports of DSM problems and Serious Theft, parent reports of DSM problems and Serious Violence, and teacher reports of DSM problems and Serious Violence are then presented sequentially.

Effects of DSM-Oriented Problems on Serious Theft and Serious Violence

In reviewing the results regarding the DSM-oriented constructs across the 24 models, some interesting findings emerge. Recall that within each individual model were four distinct DSM-oriented problems of interest. More specifically, each model tested the effect of parent and teacher reports of Oppositional Defiant Problems, Attention Deficit/Hyperactivity Problems, Anxiety Problems, and Affective Problems on Serious Theft and Serious Violence. This strategy results in a total of 96 parameter estimates consisting of four DSM problems multiplied by 24 distinct models.

When all 96 parameter estimates of these DSM effects are considered, only five out of these 96 relationships attained statistical significance at the .05 level. According to the rules of inferential statistics, we can expect that five percent, or 4.8 of these 96 possible relationships could be observed by chance. Table 7 shows that only five of the 96 total relationships reached statistical significance across the 24 regression models, hence all could have occurred by chance. Thus, when viewed within this larger picture, the argument can be made that there is an impressive *lack* of significant findings, because all of the findings could bechance occurrences and therefore not indicative of true predictive relationships across the age blocks.

Before categorically disregarding the four DSM-oriented constructs as ineffective predictors over the age blocks, however, a further deconstruction of the 24 models by type of offense shows a different possibility. That is, when looking at the 12 theft models and the 12 violence models separately, we would expect that five percent, or roughly two of the 48 (12 models x 4 coefficients per model) possible relationships, can be chance observations. When analyzed from this perspective, the findings from Table 7 indicated that only one of the 12 Serious Theft models, or Model 7 (b = .100, $se(b)$ = .049, OR = 1.106) was significant. There is, again, the possibility that this result was found at random.

When turning to the 12 violence models and the 48 possible parameter estimates for the DSM-oriented constructs, four of the 48 effects were statistically significant. As shown in the summary of findings presented in Table 7, Models 19, 20, 22, and 24 each had one significant DSM problem. Beginning with Model 19, teacher reports of Affective Problems at ages seven to nine (Age Block 1) were found to be a significant predictor of Serious Violence at Age Block 2. Thus, when controlling for other variables in the model, Affective Problems (b = .115, $se(b)$ = .046, OR = 1.122) in middle childhood were positively and significantly related to seriously violent behaviors later in childhood, with depressed boys approximately 12 percent more likely to be involved in violence. These findings remained significant throughout

Table 7 *Significant DSM-Oriented Constructs Predicting Serious Theft and Violent Behaviors for 24 Models across Informants.*

Model #	Block Y Regressed on Block X	Ages of Subjects for Blocks	Significant DSM-Oriented Constructs	Type Offense/ Informant
7	Block 2/ Block 1	10-12 years old/ 7-9 years old	Affective Problems at Age Block 1	Theft/ Teachers
19	Block 2/ Block 1	10-12 years old/ 7-9 years old	Affective Problems at Age Block 1	Violence/ Teachers
20	Block 3/ Block 1	13-16 years old/ 7-9 years old	Affective Problems at Age Block 1	Violence/ Teachers
22	Block 3/ Block 2	13-16 years old/ 10-12 years old	Attention Deficit/Hyperactivity Problems at Age Block 2	Violence/ Teachers
24	Block 4/ Block 3	17-19 years old/ 13-16 years old	Oppositional Defiant Problems at Age Block 3	Violence/ Teachers

Age Block 3 in Model 20, with Affective Problems at Age Block 1 also having a statistically significant relationship (b = .085, $se(b)$ = .038, OR = 1.089) with violent offending in PYS boys at ages 13 to 16. These effects did not remain constant throughout Age Block 4, however. Moving on to Model 22, teacher reports of Attention Deficit/Hyperactivity Problems at Age Block 2 emerged as a statistically significant predictor of Serious Violence at Age Block 3 (b = .071, $se(b)$ = .036, OR = 1.074). Again, these effects of ADHP at Age Block 2 were rendered insignificant when violence at Age Block 4 was considered.

An examination of the results in Model 24 showed that of the four mental health constructs included in the analysis, only Oppositional Defiant Problems at Age Block 3 ($b = .154$, $se(b) = .060$, $OR = 1.167$) emerged as a positive and significantly related predictor to Age Block 4 Serious Violent behaviors.

If by chance we can expect two of these four significant coefficients to be found, then the pertinent question becomes which two parameter estimates were truly significant and effective predictors of serious offending? To help clarify this research question, the results from the 24 separate logistic regressions were further scrutinized at the informant level. That is, the 24 models were first separated by offense (Serious Theft versus Serious Violence), thereby producing 12 models each. Each set of 12 models was then further divided by informant type (parents versus teachers), resulting in four subsets of six models each, and producing the subset combinations of: Parents/Serious Theft, Teachers/Serious Theft, Parents/Serious Violence, and Teachers/Serious Violence. Each of these four subsets yielded four parameter estimates of the effects of the DSM constructs, resulting in a total of 24 parameter estimates for each subgroup (six models times four estimates). At the .05 level, we can roughly approximate that one of these parameter estimates would attain significance by chance within each of the four subsets of models.

Findings across Violence and Theft Subgroups

As the findings from each subset were examined at the informant level, the robustness of the effects of the DSM-oriented constructs on future violence became more pronounced. Again, only one of the six teacher-reported DSM problems was significant for Serious Theft behaviors. Therefore, we are still left to consider that the findings from Model 7 (Serious Theft at Age Block 2 regressed on teacher reports of Affective Problems at Age Block 1) were a chance occurrence.

However, when reviewing the findings regarding the teacher-reported effects of DSM-oriented problems on Serious Violence, four of the six coefficients reached statistical significance (Models 19, 20, 22, and 24). Even when disregarding one of these parameter estimates as a chance occurrence, three statistically significant coefficients remain. Again, the question becomes which one of these four findings was observed by chance and which was truly reflective of the relationship between these DSM constructs and Serious Violence over the lifecourse?

Within a developmental or lifecourse framework, three distinct patterns of mental health problems emerge when considering the effects of the DSM-oriented constructs on future violence. First, the onset of Affective Problems in middle childhood (ages seven through nine) predicted Serious Violence in late childhood (ages 10 through 12) *and* in early adolescence (ages 13 through 16), as shown in Models 19 and 20. These findings suggest that the early onset of depression in young boys independently contributes to violent offending throughout their late adolescent years, even after controlling for all other variables within the model. These Affective Problems did not emerge as a significant predictor of violence at any other stage of childhood or adolescence.

Secondly, the effects of teacher reports of ADHP on future violence emerged as a significant predictor in late childhood only, as shown in Model 22. That is, PYS boys age 10 through 12 who had ADHP were significantly more likely to commit violent acts during early adolescence (ages 13 through 16). None of the other DSM-oriented problems reached statistical significance in late childhood for parents or teachers, and this was the only time that ADHP effects were significant for any stage of childhood or adolescence in PYS boys. Lastly, teacher-reported oppositional behaviors emerged in early adolescence (ages 13 to 16) as a significant predictor of Serious Violence in late adolescence (ages 17 through 19). Again, ODP was found to have significant effects solely for Model 24, but not for any of the other developmental periods within childhood or adolescence.

Based on the large body of literature regarding the link between ADHP and ODP and subsequent aggression, one might expect these mental health problems to both have an early and persistent onset when associated with future violence. Yet the present analysis revealed that ADHP emerged as a significant predictor of violence in late childhood (ages 10 to 12) only, with the effects of ODP not becoming significant until much later during early adolescence (ages 13 to 16). Of the two findings, the fact that ODP was not a significant predictor of violence until this late stage of development was unexpected based on the empirical evidence linking early onset childhood ODD and aggression. While it is certainly not improbable that oppositional behaviors in early adolescence could be a predictor of later violence, it was a surprise to not see these effects emerge earlier in childhood as a predictor of violence at earlier stages of development. This finding of onset of violent offending in late adolescence (ages 17 to 19) is consistent, however, within the dual taxonomy framework posited by Moffitt (1993). This theory argues that the largest numbers of youngsters will commit delinquent acts as adolescents, with offending peaking at age 17 and then dropping sharply as they emerge into young adulthood. "The majority of criminal offenders are teenagers; by the early 20s, the number of active offenders decreases by over 50 percent; and by age 28, almost 85% of former delinquents desist from offending" (Moffitt, 2001, p. 93). Thus, these findings with regard to ODP are not inconsistent with this theory of dual taxonomy, and therefore may not be spurious.

Conversely, it is possible that the significant parameter estimate of the effects of ADHP in late childhood on Serious Violence in early adolescence was also a random finding, with inconsistent conclusions throughout the literature regarding the relationship between ADHD and violence. As stated previously, while a large body of research has linked the impulsivity component of ADHD to aggression, the results have been varied with respect to the inattentive element of this disorder. Overall, however, the results here are consistent with an enormous body of scholarly literature positing that negative outcomes, such as violence and aggression, are frequently observed in children exhibiting the combined hyperactive and inattentive symptoms found within the ADHP construct during early adolescence (Connor et al., 2006). Thus, based on the available empirical literature, it appears unclear which of these two relationships could be a chance finding.

If we do consider either one of the findings related to ADHP or ODP as a possibly spurious relationship, the only remaining statistically significant effects are found in Models 19 and 20. These models both showed significant parameter estimates for the effects of Affective Problems on Serious Violence. These results stand out for several reasons. First, Affective Problems was the only DSM-oriented problem construct that had repeated significant findings across the 24 models. Secondly, both models utilized the same informant data, or teacher reports of mental health problems. These teacher reports remained consistently predictive, despite the fact that the teachers changed over the years as these children progressed in school grade.

Thirdly, it was striking that these effects emerged within the same developmental period of middle childhood, or between the ages of seven and nine years old. Thus, it appears that early depressive problems in PYS boys in middle childhood, when controlling for all other variables in the models, were significant predictors of Serious Violence during both late childhood and early adolescence, or through age 16. Lastly, the same findings regarding Affective Problem onset in middle childhood were also predictive of Serious Theft behaviors in late childhood.

Although the findings in Model 7 may admittedly be spurious, these results, at least in small part, further support the acknowledgement of depressive problems as an important predictor of serious offending behaviors over the lifecourse (see Loeber, 2004).

The overall robustness of these findings is somewhat surprising in light of the literature that would suggest that other mental health issues in childhood or adolescence would be more likely to contribute to violent behaviors in boys than Affective Problems alone. Moreover, interesting gender issues are raised by these findings with regard to the long-term impact of internalizing disorders, such as MDD and Dysthymia, on young boys as opposed to females. Even without a comorbid disruptive disorder, PYS boys were significantly more likely to commit Serious Violence in later childhood and adolescence if they were reported by their teachers to have Affective Problems.

In addition to the question of which of these significant effects may be spurious, there also exists a further need to determine how powerful these relationships are. Specifically, what is the ability of each of these five models to accurately predict future serious offending, especially when considering the normal, borderline, and clinical demarcations within the problem behavior constructs? To gauge the relative risk of either Serious Theft or Violence occurring for each of the significant mental health effects found here, the next section presents the predicted probabilities for each of these five models.

Predicted Probabilities of Significant Serious Theft and Serious Violent Models

To gain a better understanding of how well Affective Problems for boys between the ages of seven to nine predicted future serious theft behaviors, predicted probabilities were calculated for the normal, borderline, and clinical ranges of these significant DSM-oriented constructs. Recall that these constructs values were transformed from raw scores and normalized into T scores to facilitate a comparison between PYS boys and national samples of youths with the similar gender and ages. Within these probability equations, the values of the other variables besides the significant DSM-oriented problem were held at their means. A summary of these predicted probabilities is presented in Table 8 that follows.

Recall that these Affective Problem scores were censored, with normal scores truncated together beginning with a low score of 50 and ranging to a potential maximum score of 100. Normal T scores ranged from a low of 50 to a score of under 65; borderline scores ranged from 65 to under a score of 70; clinical scores ranged from a minimum score of 70 to a potential high of 100. Actual observed scores in PYS boys between the ages of seven and nine years old by teachers fell between a low score of 50 and a high score of 70.5.

To determine what the relative risk of Serious Theft was for boys in the youngest PYS sample that fell within these three ranges, the predicted probabilities for the average ($M = 55.31$), mid-borderline (67), and the highest observed scores (70.5) were each calculated for each significant DSM-oriented construct. For Model 7, these calculations suggested that boys who were in the normal/average range for Affective Problems during middle childhood had only a .068 probability of committing serious theft behaviors in late childhood. When scores increased into the borderline range (67), the risk of these behaviors increased to a .220 probability of thefts occurring. Lastly, youths scoring in the clinical level of Affective Problems (70.5) had a .312 probability of committing serious offending behaviors. Thus, this equation predicting the probabilities for theft behavior indicated an increasing, systematic progression across the three clinical cut-off scores for Affective Problems.

Table 8 *Predicted Probabilities of Significant DSM-Oriented Problem Behaviors.*

Model# Informant	DSM-Oriented Problem/ Dependent Variable	Pred Prob (Average Scores)	Pred Prob (Borderline Scores)	Pred Prob (Clinical Scores)
7 Teacher	Affective Problems/ Serious Theft	.068	.220	.312
19 Teacher	Affective Problems/ Serious Violence	.075	.290	.435
20 Teacher	Affective Problems/ Serious Violence	.161	.437	.587
22 Teacher	Att-Deficit/Hyper Prob/ Serious Violence	.180	.333	.477 (score 72) .842 (score 80)
24 Teacher	Oppositional Def Prob/ Serious Violence	.036	.292	.462

Note. Pred Prob = Predicted Probabilities. Att-Deficit/Hyper Prob = Attention Deficit/Hyperactivity Problems. Oppositional Def Prob = Oppositional Defiant Problems.

These findings suggest that there is a tangible and practical utility for distinguishing between normal, borderline, and clinical designations between boys, with the difference with normal scores of predicted probability of committing Serious Theft increasing dramatically when comparing between borderline boys with clinical levels of psychopathology. Moreover, these results point to the importance of recognizing depressive symptoms in boys in middle childhood, as they appear to influence the probability of serious theft behaviors later in the lifespan. Again, none of the other Serious Theft models had mental health constructs reach levels of statistical significance for either parent or teacher reports.

In moving back to the central issue within the present study, or the predicted probability of violence for mentally ill youths, Model 19 shows the ability of OPD, ADHP, Anxiety Problems, and Affective Problems in middle childhood (Age Block 1) in predicting Serious Violence at late childhood (Age Block 2). When controlling for other variables in the model, again only teacher reports of Affective Problems ($b = .115$, $se(b) = .046$, $OR = 1.122$) in middle childhood were positively and significantly related to seriously violent behaviors later in childhood, with depressed boys about 12 percent more likely to be involved in violent acts.

For Model 19, the same procedures were replicated to calculate the predicted probability of boys with Affective Problems at ages seven to nine committing Serious Violence between the ages of 10 and 12. When looking across these figures, Model 19 calculations determined that there was only a .075 probability of boys with average Affective scores acting violently during late childhood. However, the risk of serious antisocial behaviors began to increase dramatically as scores rose into borderline and clinical ranges. Specifically, there was a .290 and .435 probability of boys scoring at mid-borderline levels (67) or maximum observed clinical-levels (70.5) for Affective Problems between the ages seven to nine later committing seriously violent acts between the ages of 10 and 12, respectively. Again, the equation showed an increasing graduation of violent behaviors in youths across the three levels of clinical functioning for Affective Problems.

In focusing upon the teacher reports of DSM behaviors in middle childhood as a predictor of serious offending even later in the lifecourse, an examination of the logistic regression findings in Model 20 showed that the independent effects of Affective Problems continued to be a significant predictor as PYS youngsters entered early adolescence. Again, Affective Problems ($b = .085$, *se(b)* = .038, *OR* = 1.089) at Age Block 1 were a robust predictor of later violence at Age Block 3. Children who had these types of depressive problems were approximately nine percent more likely to commit Serious Violence later in their adolescence.

Moreover, the predicted probability of youths to commit violence varied dramatically when the *T* scores for Affective Problems onset in middle childhood were considered. That is, children who had normal scores for depressive problems between ages seven and nine had a .161 probability of being violent in early adolescence. By comparison, youths who had a *T* score of 67 (mid-borderline range) had a .437 probability of violence. Youths scoring at the maximum observed clinical value of just over 70 (70.5) had a .587 probability of violent behaviors between the ages of 13 and 16. These findings from Model 20 were analogous to those presented in Model 19, with the probability of future violence in youths who were reported by teachers as having borderline or clinical ranges of depression in middle childhood much greater for these boys throughout their early adolescence (Age Block 3).

Only two other models attained statistical significance for any of the mental health problems. Model 22 shows the results of Serious Violence at Age Block 3 being regressed on the teacher-reported DSM-oriented constructs at Age Block 2. When controlling for other variables in the model, Attention Deficit/Hyperactivity Problems emerged for the first time as having a positive and significant effect on Serious Violence for PYS boys in early adolescence. Recall that youths with ADHD had truncated *T* scores such that the minimum possible score started at a low score of 50 and ranged to a maximum score possible of 80.

When converted to predicted probabilities, the impact of ADH Problems became even more evident. As with the other statistically significant models, boys with normal, borderline, and clinical *T* scores were distinct from one another when considering their propensity to commit violent acts. These analyses indicated that PYS boys with average teacher reported ADHP scores (*M* = 58.46) in late childhood had a .180 predicted probability of acting violently in early adolescence. Comparatively, a dramatic rise in these values was observed as boys moved from borderline *T* scores toward maximum clinical scores. That is, for boys with mid-borderline levels of ADHP (67), there was a .333 probability of Serious Violence at Age Block 3. For PYS youths scoring within a low clinical range (72) and maximum observed clinical scores (80) between the ages of 10 and 12, the probabilities of seriously violent behavior between the ages of 13 and 16 climbed from .477 to .842, respectively. Therefore, this equation indicated that boys with borderline or clinical scores of ADHP had impressive predicted probabilities for violent acts when compared to boys within normal ranges. As such, boys having either borderline or low clinical ADHP scores in late childhood had considerably greater chances of committing violent behaviors in later childhood.

Model 24 presents the final significant teacher model regarding the ability of DSM-oriented mental health problems to predict Serious Violence in late adolescence. Of the four mental health constructs included in the analysis, only Oppositional Defiant Problems at Age Block 3 emerged as a positive and significant predictor of Age Block 4 Serious Violent behaviors. Recall that these scores for Oppositional Defiant Problems ranged from low *T* scores of 50 to maximum clinical scores of 75.

Again, predicted probabilities were calculated for the average score within the youngest sample (*M* = 58.56), as well as for mid-borderline (67), and the maximum observed clinical score (75). These calculations indicated that the probability of violent behaviors in late adolescence (Age

Block 4) increased significantly between these three scores, such that youths with normal average ODP scores had only a .036 probability of Serious Violence between the ages of 17 and 19. In contrast to this quite modest estimate, PYS adolescents between the ages of 13 and 16 with either borderline or clinical ranges of Oppositional Defiant Problems were at much greater risk of committing violent acts, with the probability of antisocial violent behavior in these boys calculated at .292 and .462, respectively. Just as seen in previous equations, then, the predicted probability of violence in youths with graduating progressions of ODP across the three cut-off scores increased significantly as youths moved away from normal scores. From this perspective, it appears that the presence of teacher-reported oppositional problems in early adolescence drastically increased the likelihood of serious violence later in the lifecourse.

For all boys with borderline levels of significant mental health problems, the greatest probability of violence (.437) came from youths who were reported by their teachers to have Affective Problems in middle childhood as a predictor of Serious Violence in early adolescence. With regard to PYS boys who reached clinical levels of mental health dysfunction, youngsters with Affective Problems in middle childhood had an impressive .587 probability of committing Serious Violence in early adolescence. Boys in late childhood who reached clinical scores of Attention-Deficit/Hyperactivity Problems were even more likely to commit Serious Violence in their early adolescence, with a .477 probability for youths with a T score of 70.5 and a .842 probability of violence for ADHP youths assigned the maximum possible clinical score of 80. Unquestionably, this summary highlights the strength of these forms of childhood and adolescent psychopathology in predicting later serious offending behaviors. Now that the significant results with regard to the DSM-oriented problems have been examined, the effects of the controls included within these models are briefly explored.

Control Variable Effects on Serious Theft Behaviors

To ease in interpretation and understanding of the numerous models presented in Appendixes F through Q, Table 9 summarizes the statistically significant variables for each of the 12 Serious Theft models. All of the statistically significant variables for each of these models are listed for the reader. This presentation allows for a global perspective of the significant effects of all independent variables while controlling for other variables in the model. As discussed in the previous methods chapter, this study was designed to be sensitive to critics who have argued that developmentally-oriented studies using psychologically-based measures are tautological in nature because they do not adequately control for previous delinquent behaviors. Both the temporal design of the age blocks and the inclusion of previous Serious Theft and Serious Violence in each model attempts to control for omitted variables that may be a source of spuriousness.

As Serious Theft is the first dependent variable of interest, the statistically significant results for the 12 parent and teacher models are presented first in Table 9 (see Appendixes F through Q for all tables). As expected, the most consistent significant effect was the existence of serious theft behaviors in the age block most proximal to that of the dependent variable age block. Importantly, Serious Theft behaviors at Age Block 1 (ages seven to nine) were unavailable for two of these 12 models, or Models 1 and 7. However, the remaining 10 models each yielded significant findings that theft behaviors at the previous age block were a significant predictor of theft behaviors within the age block of the dependent variable. These control effects were quite robust, with the likelihood of those boys with prior Serious Theft behaviors of committing similar thefts in the next age block ranging from a low of nine times (Models 2, 4, and 10) to a high of more than 15 times (Model 6).

Table 9 *Statistically Significant Variables across 12 Serious Theft Models from Parent and Teacher Reports.*

Model #	Block Y Regressed on Block X	Ages of Subjects for Blocks	Significant Variables in Model	Informant
1	Block 2/Block 1	10-12 years old/ 7-9 years old	None	Parents
2	Block 3/Block 1	13-16 years old/ 7-9 years old	Serious Theft at Age Block 2 Serious Violence at Age Block 2 Low Family SES at Age Block 2	Parents
3	Block4/Block 1	17-19 years old/ 7-9 years old	Serious Theft at Age Block 3 Race	Parents
4	Block 3/Block 2	13-16 years old/ 10-12 years old	Serious Theft at Age Block 2 Serious Violence at Age Block 2	Parents
5	Block 4/Block 2	17-19 years old/ 10-12 years old	Serious Theft at Age Block 3 Race	Parents
6	Block 4/Block 3	17-19 years old/ 13-16 years old	Serious Theft at Age Block 3 Race	Parents
7	Block 2/Block 1	10-12 years old/ 7-9 years old	Affective Problems at Age Block 1	Teachers

Continued on next page

Table 9 continued

Model #	Block Y Regressed on Block X	Ages of Subjects for Blocks	Significant Variables in Model	Informant
8	Block 3/Block 1	13-16 years old/ 7-9 years old	Serious Theft at Age Block 2 Serious Violence at Age Block 2	Teachers
9	Block 4/Block 1	17-19 years old/ 7-9 years old	Serious Theft at Age Block 3 Race	Teachers
10	Block 3/Block 2	13-16 years old/ 10-12 years old	Serious Theft at Age Block 2	Teachers
11	Block 4/Block 2	17-19 years old/ 10-12 years old	Serious Theft at Age Block 3 Race	Teachers
12	Block 4/Block 3	17-19 years old/ 13-16 years old	Serious Theft at Age Block 3 Low Family SES at Age Block 2 Race	Teachers

Three other controls were also outstanding predictors of Serious Theft across the 12 models. First, race had significant negative effects in half of the theft models, with three models each significant for parents and teachers (see Models 3, 5, 6, 9, 11, and 12, respectively). That is, for each of these six models, blacks were significantly less likely to commit Serious Theft than were whites. The odds ratios of these control effects were quite modest overall, however.

Not surprisingly, youths who committed Serious Violence at the most proximal age block to the one of the dependent variable were also significantly more likely to commit Serious Theft in three of the 12 theft models (Models 2, 4, and 8). The sizes of the odds ratios for previous acts of violence were not as large as those seen in the Serious Theft controls. Indeed, these youths were approximately three times as likely to commit Serious Theft for each of the significant parameter estimates within these models.

The last control variable to have any predictive ability on Serious Theft offending was Family SES, with youngsters coming from families in the lowest quartile (Low Family SES) significantly more likely to commit theft behaviors in Models 2 and 12. Boys between the ages of 10 and 12 who came from families with lower SES were roughly two times (in early adolescence) and five times more likely (in late adolescence) to commit Serious Theft behaviors, respectively.

In sum, then, the most dominant control variable emerging across these 12 Serious Theft models was the presence of Serious Theft in the time period closest to that of the dependent variable in the model. This finding is not startling and should also be germane when considering the proximity of earlier violent behaviors on the future prediction of violence as a control variable. The results from these violence models are examined in the section that follows.

Control Variable Effects on Serious Violence Behaviors

Of the two dependent variables in the analysis, Serious Violence is admittedly the more important from a criminological standpoint and with regard to implications. Table 10 offers the reader a summary of the statistically significant control variables across the 12 Serious Violence models (see Appendixes F through Q for a complete presentation of findings). A review of these findings revealed very similar patterns to those discussed in the Serious Theft models with respect to previous offending behaviors. That is, of all the significant control variable effects found across these models, previous acts of violence emerged as the most consistent predictor of future violence, with *all* models reporting significant coefficients. Indeed, boys who either self-reported or had official records for Physical Aggression or Serious Violence in the age block closest to that of the dependent variable were roughly three to five times more likely to commit violence again across the developmental age blocks.

Comparable to the findings regarding the Serious Violence control effects within the Serious Theft models, previous thefts were also robust predictors of Serious Violence across eight of the 12 models. Again, no previous theft reports were available for the two models at Age Block 1 (Models 13 and 19). Thus, five of the parent models (Models 14, 15, 16, 17, and 18) and three of the teacher models (Models 21, 22, and 23) had statistically significant parameter estimates of previous theft effects on later violent acts. Specifically, boys who had previous reports for Serious Theft previously were roughly five times more likely to commit Serious Violence across these models. These findings were not surprising due to the strong body of literature that suggests that there is great heterogeneity in offending throughout childhood and adolescence (Piquero & Mazerolle, 2001).

Table 10 *Statistically Significant Variables across 12 Serious Violence Models from Parent and Teacher Reports.*

Model #	Block Y Regressed on Block X	Ages of Subjects for Blocks	Significant Variables in Model	Informant
13	Block 2/Block 1	10-12 years old/ 7-9 years old	Physical Aggression at Age Block 1 Race	Parents
14	Block 3/Block 1	13-16 years old/ 7-9 years old	Serious Violence at Age Block 2 Serious Theft at Age Block 2 Race	Parents
15	Block4/Block 1	17-19 years old/ 7-9 years old	Serious Violence at Age Block 3 Serious Theft at Age Block 3 Typical Family SES at Age Block 1	Parents
16	Block 3/Block 2	13-16 years old/ 10-12 years old	Serious Violence at Age Block 2 Serious Theft at Age Block 2 Low Family SES at Age Block 2 Race	Parents
17	Block 4/Block 2	17-19 years old/ 10-12 years old	Serious Violence at Age Block 3 Serious Theft at Age Block 3 Typical Family SES at Age Block 1 Race	Parents

Continued on next page

Table 10 continued

Model #	Block Y Regressed on Block X	Ages of Subjects for Blocks	Significant Variables in Model	Informant
18	Block 4/Block 3	17-19 years old/ 13-16 years old	Serious Violence at Age Block 3 Serious Theft at Age Block 3 Typical Family SES at Age Block 1 Race	Parents
19	Block 2/Block 1	10-12 years old/ 7-9 years old	Affective Problems at Age Block 1 Physical Aggression at Age Block 1	Teachers
20	Block 3/Block 1	13-16 years old/ 7-9 years old	Affective Problems at Age Block 1 Serious Violence at Age Block 2	Teachers
21	Block 4/Block 1	17-19 years old/ 7-9 years old	Serious Violence at Age Block 3 Serious Theft at Age Block 3 Typical Family SES at Age Block 1	Teachers
22	Block 3/Block 2	13-16 years old/ 10-12 years old	Attention Deficit/Hyperactivity Problems at Age Block 2 Serious Violence at Age Block 2 Serious Theft at Age Block 2	Teachers
23	Block 4/Block 2	17-19 years old/ 10-12 years old	Serious Violence at Age Block 3 Serious Theft at Age Block 3 Typical Family SES at Age Block 1	Teachers

Table 10 continued

24	Block 4/Block 3	17-19 years old/ 13-16 years old	Oppositional Defiant Problems at Age Block 3 Serious Violence at Age Block 3 Typical Family SES at Age Block 1	Teachers

Family SES next emerged as a prominent and robust predictive control variable in these models, albeit with some notable exceptions to those found within the Serious Theft models discussed previously. That is, whereas only two of the 12 Serious Theft models showed Low Family SES as significantly related to future theft behaviors, only Model 16 reported Low Family SES as a significant variable within the Serious Violence models. Accordingly, those boys with Low Family SES at Age Block 2 (ages 10 through 12) were over two times more likely to commit violence in Age Block 3. In comparison, Typical Family SES at Age Block 1 (ages seven through nine) emerged as a robust and consistent predictor across a majority of the remaining violence models, with six of the 11 models reporting significant effects for this control variable (Models 15, 17, 18, 21, 23, and 24, respectively). The odds ratios for these models revealed that youths with Typical Family SES scores (in between the lowest and highest quartiles) were roughly four to six times more likely to commit serious violence within the six models.

With regard to race, some critical differences were found when the results from the Serious Theft models were compared to the Serious Violence models. Although blacks were found to be significantly *less* likely to commit Serious Theft behaviors in six of the 12 models, an opposite race effect was found when looking at Serious Violence as the dependent variable. Specifically, in five of the 12 models (Models 13, 14, 16, 17, and 18), blacks were significantly *more* likely to commit violence. Notably, however, none of these significant race effects emerged from teacher reports, where the statistically significant mental health problems were found. Nonetheless, blacks in these five models were all between two and three times more likely to commit violence than were whites within the sample.

Summary of Results

Similar to the trends for the control variables found within the Serious Theft models, a review of the findings for these 12 Serious Violence models revealed that previous violence emerged as the most consistent significant effect of future violent behavior. When including Physical Aggression, all 12 Serious Violence models reported that violent behaviors in the age block just prior to that of the dependent variable were significant and robust predictors of future violence.

When moving away from the control variables and back to the focus of this research, or the ability of ODP, ADHP, Anxiety, and Affective Problems to predict serious offending behaviors in children and adolescents, the results of these analyses show some clear developmental patterns that require further thought. These findings clearly highlight the significance of specific mental health problems at various develop-mental periods across childhood and adolescence as robust predictors of Serious Violence in particular.

CHAPTER 5

Implications and Conclusions

This study had the benefit of using data from one of the preeminent longitudinal datasets in the world—the Pittsburgh Youth Study. For approximately twenty years, Rolf Loeber and his colleagues have collected prospective data across a multitude of instruments from boys, parents, and teachers. The methodological contributions of the PYS make it one of the richest datasets for researchers to use in the investigation of the temporal relationships between individual, family, and neighborhood level indicators and poor lifecourse outcomes. The current study has several methodological advantages worth mentioning at the outset.

First, few data sets currently exist that offer the low attrition rate, prospective design, number of measurements, assortment of instruments, and regularity in assessments as those found within the PYS. Secondly, the large sample size and multiple informants provided prospective data from preadolescent youths, parents, and teachers. Thirdly, the combination of youth self-reports and official reports of offending behaviors within the dependent variables allowed for a more comprehensive picture of offending within the sample than relying on one data source (Piquero & Mazerolle, 2001; Achenbach, 2006).

The intentional oversampling of "at-risk" youths and their families within the PYS in itself produced important findings. When the figures regarding parent and teacher reports of mental health problems are combined with knowledge about the oversampling of "at-risk" youths inherent in the design of the PYS, one might expect that PYS boys would have greater levels of offending than other youngsters nationally. A review of these descriptive statistics, however, revealed that PYS youths levels of offending were actually comparable to reports throughout the academic literature, with PYS boys committing theft and violence infrequently during late childhood, increasing criminal acts in early adolescence, and then largely desisting in these behaviors during late adolescence. These rates of theft and violence in PYS youths were analogous to previous studies on rates of juvenile offending (Farrington, 1986; Sampson & Laub, 2001; see also Fabio et al., 2006).

Summary of Key Findings

The primary goal of this study was to determine the "reach" of selected childhood and adolescent mental health problems in the prediction of serious offending behaviors throughout childhood and adolescence (see Loeber, 2004). Toward this end, the present study tested 24 logistic regression models to determine the role of parent and teacher reports of ODP, ADHP, Anxiety Problems, and Affective Problems (from middle childhood throughout early adolescence) in the prediction of Serious Theft and Serious Violence (from late childhood throughout late adolescence). While the primary focus of this study centered around the prediction of violence, serious theft behaviors were included here to allow for comparisons between the pathways of different types of serious offending behaviors. These findings were mired and complex.

To help synthesize these key findings of this study, four of the main points are briefly discussed below, including: 1) the predictive value of the DSM-oriented constructs, 2) the utility of making distinctions across varying levels of mental health dysfunction, 3) the prominence of teacher reports as effective informants, and 4) the importance of the Family SES and race effects that emerged when looking across the models.

Effectiveness of Various Indicators in Predicting Violence

Accordingly, this discussion now turns toward exploring the results with regard to the first two primary findings: 1) the effectiveness of different mental health indicators at varying stages of childhood and adolescence in predicting serious violence over the lifecourse, *and* 2) the practical utility of making distinctions between normal, borderline, and clinical levels of psychological problems in youngsters. Working together within a developmental framework, both of these items make important contributions to our understanding of the complex relationship between mental health and serious juvenile offending.

Recall the four models that predicted Serious Violence. The first key finding is that three different teacher-reported DSM-oriented problems, originating in three different developmental periods, significantly predicted later violent acts. Sequentially, PYS boys with Affective Problems in middle childhood had a significantly greater likelihood of committing Serious Violence in both the late childhood *and* early adolescence. Next, youths with an onset of Attention-Deficit/Hyperactivity Problems during late childhood were significantly more likely to commit violent acts during their early adolescence. Lastly, young males in their early adolescent years with Oppositional Defiant Problems were more likely to act violently in late adolescence.

In addition to prediction, a noteworthy caveat within these findings is that they suggest the direction of the causal relationships between mental health and antisocial acts. These results suggest that mental health was temporally predictive of serious violence later in the lifecourse, while simultaneously controlling for previous criminal acts, SES, and race. Such issues are of critical

concern for developmental and lifecourse researchers today
(Loeber, 2004).

In sum, while the presence of Affective Problems was
an important mental health issue in middle childhood, they
were not predictive of violence in other stages of childhood
or adolescence. The same conclusions can be drawn for
both ADHP and ODP, with each having significant effects
at differing developmental periods in PYS boys. These
findings have serious implications with regard to the
temporal role of mental illness in the etiology of violence,
especially because these variables attained statistical
significance when controlling for previous theft and
violence, Family SES, and race.

Contributions of DSM-Oriented Scales

The second main point refers to the methodological
contribution of using DSM-oriented scales to measure
various forms of mental health dysfunction, as opposed to
the categorical diagnoses found within the DSM. Due to
the dichotomous nature of DSM diagnoses, these categories
do not allow for consideration of the effects of borderline
psychiatric problems that fail to meet a clinical threshold.
In contrast, the DSM-oriented constructs used within the
present study offer a relatively new and innovative
measurement technique to gauge the causal relationships of
these mental health problems with subsequent offending
behaviors in PYS youths. By also calculating the predicted
probability of violence for the significant DSM-oriented
problems, these results showed the utility of simultaneously
predicting future violence while also making clinical
distinctions between levels of mental health dysfunction.

To briefly restate these findings across the four models
that predicted Serious Violence, boys within normal ranges
of DSM-oriented problems had very modest probabilities
of committing later violent acts when compared to youths
with either borderline or clinical teacher reports of mental
health dysfunction. For example, while boys with

borderline levels of Affective Problems in middle childhood had a .437 probability of committing Serious Violence in their late childhood, youths within normal ranges for depressive problems were found to have only a .161 probability of acting violently. The probability of violence in these PYS youths continued to increase dramatically as scores progressed into clinical levels of psychopathology, with depressed boys having a .587 probability of violence in late childhood.

The robustness of these predictive probabilities was not unique to this model; it was a constant throughout the four significant Serious Violence models. Indeed, the most impressive probability to emerge was found when comparing between normal, borderline, and clinical levels of ADHP. Whereas boys with normal scores for ADH problems in late childhood had only a .180 probability of violence in early adolescence, youths within borderline ranges of these problems had a .333 probability of acting violently. Even more impressive was the strength of these estimates in predicting violence for juveniles assigned within clinical ranges, with boys at a low-clinical and maximum-clinical score having a .477 and .842 predicted probability of violence, respectively. Undoubtedly, such distinctions across normal, borderline, and clinical levels of mental health dysfunction found within these DSM-oriented constructs offer researchers a powerful predictive tool when considering patterns of systematic progression toward violence.

Moreover, while the decision to employ these DSM-oriented scales was made primarily because they offered these clinical distinctions, an additional benefit was that they allowed for comparisons between PYS youths and national samples by converting raw scores to *T* scores. Such a review was previously unavailable. An examination revealed that PYS boys had higher means for teacher reports of OPD, ADHP, Anxiety, and Affective Problems when weighed against national samples.

Parent versus Teacher Reports of Psychopathology

A third key finding here highlights the prominence of teachers as effective informants of child mental health dysfunction. Parent and teacher reports of psychopathology were remarkably different. It was striking that none of the mental health problems attained statistical significance across any of the 12 parent models. In contrast, five of these 12 teacher models examining mental health relationships with serious theft or violence were significant.

Some noticeable differences also became apparent when looking within and across the teacher models. Overall, only one of the six teacher models was significant for Serious Theft. Therefore, four of the six Serious Violence models had significant findings for at least one of the teacher-reported mental health problems. These findings indicate that teachers were more objective reporters than parents of significant forms of childhood and adolescent psychopathology that predicted serious offending behaviors, especially violence.

These comparisons between parents and teachers highlight an important methodological strength within the PYS study design, with repeated data collections from multiple informants. The salience of comparing reports of problem behaviors between informant sources has been well accepted within developmental psychology for some time now (Achenbach, 1985; Duhig, Renk, Epstein, & Phares, 2000). Varying levels of functioning are typically observed across these different domains (e.g., home and school), thus making such comparisons between informants a valuable tool when investigating serious offending behaviors.

Without a doubt, there are negative connotations associated with the assignment of symptoms for mental health problems, regardless of the informant. Following this logic, it stands to reason that parents may mitigate their child's behaviors because they may view these problems as reflective of their own dysfunction or failure in parenting. Conversely, educators may be more objective informants of childhood or adolescent psychological functioning given their professional training and personal distance (Kline & Silver, 2004). In sum, the results here provide further empirical support for the necessity to design studies with the ability to compare across domains and informants. Such studies offer the best chance of tackling the complex nature of how problem behaviors may impact varying types of offending behaviors over the lifecourse.

Significant Control Variables

Lastly, several key findings with regard to the Family SES and race control variables are explored in turn. Recall that the Family SES measure was computed using the Hollingshead index of social status. This measure approximated the top and bottom 25th percentiles and separated these groups from the families placing in the middle 50th, thereby creating a trichotomized variable (Low, Typical, and High Family SES).

Taken as a whole, the significant SES effects that emerged across these models appear surprising in light of prior research. In contrast to expectations, Low Family SES had little effect overall on offending behaviors, with only two of the Serious Theft models and one of the Serious Violence models reporting significant coefficients. These findings appear to contradict studies that have shown factors associated with lower socioeconomic status, or downward social mobility, high-crime neighborhoods, availability of public assistance, a lack of financial resources, and parental psychopathology, were negatively related to antisocial behaviors (Harnish, Dodge, & Valente, 1995; Lahey, Miller, Gordon, & Riley, 1999). Such poor economic standing has been shown to undermine the ability of families to seek out mental health services for themselves or their children (Miech, Caspi, Moffitt, Wright, & Silva, 1999; Kilgore, Snyder, & Lentz, 2000).

The emergence of Typical Family SES as a significant predictor of violence in half of the 12 Serious Violence models also appeared odd. Youths coming from families in this middle 50 percent of Family SES were significantly more likely to engage in violent behaviors within six of these models. These Typical SES effects were quite robust, such that these youths were approximately four to six times more likely to commit violence.

One possible explanation for these findings is that the Hollingshead SES measure may simply be distinguishing between *degrees* of disadvantage in underprivileged, inner-city, at-risk families from within Pittsburgh. This theory is a plausible one, as families within this Typical SES category were only "typical" when compared to other families participating in the PYS. Obviously, the quartiling of the Family SES measure is not an equivalent to national means for low, typical, and high SES. Thus, these categories cannot be compared to families with "typical" financial means found within national samples. Future analyses may want to include alternate measures of socioeconomic status, such as female-headed households, welfare, and/or public assistance measures, which could help to shed more light on these findings.

Similarly, some interesting findings also emerged when considering race. Recall that race was measured in the PYS using a dichotomous variable, with just over half the respondents being black (58%) and less than half being white (42%). Whites were defined as persons of European or Asian ancestry. Blacks were broadly defined as persons of African, Hispanic, American Indian, or mixed ancestry.

With regard to race differences within the analyses, an inverse pattern emerged when looking across the models. More specifically, whites were significantly more likely than blacks to commit Serious Theft offenses in six of these 12 models, with three models each for parents and teachers. Such findings were not entirely surprising because other researchers have found supporting evidence of race-ethnicity differences when looking across various types of criminal offending (Blum et al., 2000).

However, these findings were in stark contrast to the race effects on violence, such that black youths were significantly more likely to act violently within five of the 12 Serious Violence models. Furthermore, all of these effects came from parent reports. In other words, none of these significant race effects emerged from teacher reports, where the statistically significant mental health problems were found.

Thus, while blacks were significantly more likely to commit violence in five of the six parent models, caution should be used in interpreting the meaning of these findings. A potential confounding issue here is the combination of both African American and Hispanic youths within the "black" category. Future inquiries may want to consider further separating these racial and ethnic groups to provide a clearer picture of this relationship between race and violence. Such a disaggregation may also help determine if these effects are an artifact of negative peer or gang influences, as recent studies have reported that whites were less likely than African American or Hispanic boys to join delinquent gangs (Lahey et al., 1999).

Despite any limitations with the race variable, these findings point to a salient problem within African American and Hispanic communities that is largely consistent with prior studies. These populations have a disproportionate risk of offending and incarceration, with recent studies on first incarceration rates projecting that 32 percent of African American and 17 percent of Hispanic men will become incarcerated in their lifetimes, as compared to less than six percent of whites (U.S. Bureau of Justice Statistics, 2006). This corresponds to roughly one out of every three African American men being under some form of correctional control in the United States if current rates of first incarceration are maintained. Under the present crime control model of justice that dominates American corrections and law enforcement efforts, these figures highlight the crisis facing minority communities. As such, the findings here underscore the need for greater prevention and intervention efforts to lower the large numbers of minority youths entering the criminal justice system or becoming victims of violence.

In conclusion, the first main points presented here spotlighted the ability of specific childhood and adolescent mental health problems to predict types of serious offending behaviors in juveniles. Secondly, the adoption of the DSM-oriented scales allowed for meaningful estimations regarding the probability of serious theft and violence in youngsters with sub-threshold and clinical levels of psychopathological problems. Thirdly, the availability of parent and teacher reports from the PYS allowed for valuable cross-informant comparisons. Finally, although several SES and race effects emerged, these findings need to be viewed cautiously. With these key points examined, the discussion next explores the substantive implications of these findings.

Substantive Implications Regarding Depression

This study has enormous substantive implications as they relate to: 1) depression, 2) teacher-related labeling processes, and 3) lifecourse theories of development. In looking at the first substantive topic, one of the more robust findings to emerge across the teacher models related to the ability of Affective Problems in middle childhood to predict Serious Violence. As summarized previously, boys with depressive problems between the ages of seven and nine were significantly more likely to commit violent acts throughout early adolescence, or ages 13 to 16. These results are not easily dismissed, as they were the only mental health construct that had repeated predictive value across the violence models.

Depression is a serious health concern that puts these youngsters at elevated risk for future depression and suicide (Fergusson, Horwood, Ridder, & Beautrais, 2005).

Although the presence of depression nationally is roughly equal for prepubescent boys and girls (Kline & Silver, 2004), affective disorders may receive little attention when co-occurring with other disruptive behaviors known to commonly accompany depressive symptoms in males (Cochran & Rabinowitz, 2000; Fong, Frost, & Stansfeld, 2001). Indeed, a large body of literature has found that boys displayed externalizing behaviors as a manifestation of their depression, whereby they "expressed their unhappiness directly, angrily, and without hesitation by acting out on the world" (Gjerde, 1995, p. 1278). Other researchers have suggested that there is a "hidden depression" in males that accounts for their overrepresentation in violent acts over the lifecourse (Brownhill, Wilhelm, Barclay, & Schmied, 2005). Fromm (1973) theorized in his seminal work *The Anatomy of Human Destructiveness* that chronic boredom and depression was frequently at the root of acts of violence, including those that appeared senseless.

In addition, there may be a reciprocal relationship that emerges between the onset of depressive symptoms and violence that might reinforce these behaviors. It is expected that depressed boys might act withdrawn, aggressive, or recalcitrant in their disposition. They may fail to meet their potential for academic performance within school, miss deadlines, and feel that they are a disappointment to their teachers and parents. Long-term outcomes with employment and educational opportunities typically suffer, thereby reinforcing negative feelings within these boys. As their frustration and depression with their perceived failures grows, they could continue to act out aggressively and further escalate criminal behaviors, which would in turn only further perpetuate their depressive state and disconnect the youth from prosocial family members, educators, and peers.

For teachers, then, the violent behaviors they may witness in the school setting may actually be masking the real problem within these youths, or depression, as these findings suggest. When teachers are faced with dealing with the overtly aggressive or violent externalizing behaviors likely to be observed in these boys, it is possible that the underlying reasons driving these behaviors may be lost. Simply put, some youths may have a multitude of factors that could be expected to lead to depression in many individuals.

The source of the significant depressive effects reported here might be reflective of the micro-level impact of crime control policies that created record numbers of male minorities under some form of correctional control beginning in the 1990s. Throughout urban minority and disadvantaged communities across America, families and youths face considerable challenges on social, economic, and structural levels. Incarceration rates have been staggering in particular for African American males throughout urban communities, with estimates of 1 in 3 being under some form of correctional control nationally. In addition, many of these families must also cope with , to being at increased risk of both victimization and offending, as well as other serious social problems such as family disruptions, poverty, chronic stress from decreased social and economic mobility, high rates of alcohol and substance abuse, child maltreatment and neglect, increased risks of acute medical infections, and the negative influence of gang and community violence (Rudolph, Hammen & Daley, 2006; Lien, Haavet, Thoresen, Heyerdahl, & Bjertness, 2007)).

Increasingly, more studies have begun to look at the debilitating affects of depression earlier in the lifecourse (see van Lang, Ferdinand, & Verhulst, 2007). One recent work showed that specific traits such as fearfulness and frustration were significantly related to depression in preadolescents (Oldehinkel, Hartman, de Winter, Veenstra, & Ormel, 2004). The present findings may offer peripheral support for these previous works since these children are likely to experience significant fear and anxiety over the environmental and familial situations they face daily. Such societal conditions clearly impact youths and need to be addressed as early as possible. If society pathologizes youth without examining the contributing factors, we risk that our interventions will have limited effects on substantially reducing youth violence.

These considerations are important not just on a substantive level, but also have significant meaning with regard to treatment and identification of depressed boys. The appropriate treatment modalities for these children (and their families) continues to be a source of considerable controversy in the mental health field. It is well recognized that "depression is a major health problem, causing high societal costs and severe individual suffering and disability" (Oldehinkel, Veenstra, Ormel, de Winter, & Verhulst, 2006, p. 684). Boys with depressive problems may display paranoid, delusional, restlessness, impulsive, and poor interpersonal skills that put them at risk of continuing on with antisocial behaviors, including violence. Studies have shown that the treatment of depressive symptoms, especially in aggressive youths, is an important step in moving these children toward prosocial attitudes and behaviors (Boesky, 2005).

The availability and interest of parents in adopting and promoting treatment solutions within these families is a critical point if we are to be successful in identifying children who are not coping well to social stressors. Many of these youngsters included in this sample come from dysfunctional, at-risk, and/or highly stressed familial environments. Thus, while these findings need to be replicated with other populations and longitudinal data, it is quite possible that early intervention efforts on the part of teachers and educational personnel, especially when combined with active and promotive parenting, might prevent future serious violent offending in youths with Affective Problems.

Substantive Implications of Labeling

Secondly, the significance of teacher reports of DSM-oriented problems may be indicative of an age-graded labeling process occurring within educational settings. As schools serve as the *de facto* mental health care system for treating child mental health problems (Burns et al., 1995; Leaf et al., 1996), the findings here of teacher reports of forms of psychopathology could be an artifact of the training and sensitivity of educators in identifying hyperactive and disruptive behaviors in their classrooms. Such behavioral labels of mental health dysfunction may be passed informally between teachers as educators discuss emotional issues or problems with certain students, thereby passing on this label to teachers at other grade levels (Kline & Silver, 2004). Therefore, it could be that teachers are employing labeling of certain types of behaviors at certain developmental age periods.

Similar to criminological labeling theory, which posits that contact with the criminal justice system leads to increased internal and external stigmatization (Lemert, 1951; 1967), students may begin to internalize these teacher-assigned labels, thereby reinforcing negative psychopathological behaviors across stages of child development and grade levels. This labeling process might begin with teachers identifying a surly, difficult, or oppositional child that stands out amongst their peers in the classroom. While the teacher may take steps to address the problem behaviors, the child may begin to resent or act out against being treated "differently" than other students. It would not be unusual for teachers to discuss these frustrations and challenges with their colleagues, thereby transferring their "label" of the student. Such a process could easily have a negative impact on children and create a self-fulfilling prophesy for children labeled with serious mental health issues. Following this logic, and fueled by the present-day concerns with overcrowding, strained resources, and the threat of violence within our schools, it stands to reason that teachers may advertently or inadvertently label "problem" children to conserve time, minimize disruptions, and maintain safety.

Although the possibility of such labeling effects is worth mention here, this option does not exclude the consideration of more criminologically-oriented explanations for these results. Specifically, it is argued here that these findings may be a product of a lifecourse age-graded/developmental sequencing of problem behaviors as they impact future serious offending. There is compelling evidence here to support such a lifecourse orientation. Three different mental health problems emerged across three distinct stages of childhood and adolescent development and predicted two types of offending, or serious theft and violence.

Substantive Implications Related to Lifecourse Research

The present findings are consistent, at least to a preliminary extent, with existing lifecourse theories of antisocial behavior. For example, Moffitt's theory of dual taxonomy (1993) posits that two typologies of offenders exist: adolescence-limited (AL) and life-course-persistent (LCP). These AL offenders typically commit relatively minor property or status offenses and seldom act violently, with the first onset of delinquent behaviors around the period of puberty (Jeglum-Bartusch, Lynam, Moffitt, & Silva, 1997). These youths tend to commit delinquent behaviors due to the influence of peer pressure and are not naturally inclined to commit serious antisocial behaviors as they progress on into adulthood and adopt more conventional roles within society (Moffitt et al., 2002; Piquero & Moffitt, 2005).

In contrast, LCP offenders make up a small group within society, accounting for roughly five to eight percent of the population (Piquero & Moffitt, 2005). These persons tend to display early onset and persistence, commit a disproportionate amount of crime, and exhibit persistent heterogeneity in their offense types. This "heterotypic continuity" in LCP offending patterns, which are committed sequentially and at various stages of development, contributes to the understanding of the function of antisocial offending for these individuals (Piquero & Moffitt, 2005). These youthful offenders are more likely to commit violence, act alone, and continue with antisocial and criminal behaviors throughout adulthood (Moffitt, 1993; Jeglum-Bartusch et al., 1997; Moffitt et al., 2002). Most salient to the present findings, these youngsters' "risk for life-course-persistent offending emerges from inherited or acquired neuro-psychological variation, initially manifested as subtle cognitive defects, difficult temperament, or hyperactivity" (Piquero & Moffitt, 2005, p. 53).

The findings of depressive, oppositional, and attention-deficit/hyperactive behaviors in violent PYS boys lends some support to previous studies reporting neuro-psychological and behavioral problems within LCP offenders (Moffitt, Lynam, & Silva, 1994). However, it is outside the scope of the present study to determine if PYS boys with these DSM-oriented problems fit within an AL or LCP taxonomy. These analyses do not identify the frequency of criminal acts, track within-individual changes in the types of offenses committed, or determine the continuity of mental health problems. Such issues certainly warrant further consideration.

Public Policy Implications

Although the results presented here provide strong evidence of the negative consequences that specific mental health problems may play in the temporal development of serious offending, these findings must be interpreted with great care. Admittedly, this study is exploratory in nature and these findings are far from conclusive. Moreover, it is important to note that the vast majority of the DSM-oriented problems within these models failed to attain statistical significance. Taken as a whole, five of the 96 possible mental health problems relationships were predictive of either Serious Theft or Serious Violence. Therefore, while a clear pattern was observed when looking across the five significant models of mental health problems, the presence of many other forms of psychopathology had no statistically significant relationships with serious juvenile offending. With these limitations being understood, the significant findings that were observed here make it necessary to critically assess what public policy implications can be inferred from this study.

Serious juvenile offending is an important topic within criminology and one that has direct public policy implications for prevention and intervention efforts (Dembo, Williams et al., 1990; Loeber et al., 1998; Dembo et al., 1999; Kempf-Leonard et al., 2001; Heide, 2003; Boesky, 2002), particularly for at-risk and disadvantaged youths (Tarnowski & Blechman, 1991; Loeber & Farrington, 1998; Boesky, 2002; Heitmeyer & Hagan, 2003). Recent studies show that an increasing number of juvenile offenders have serious mental health problems, with few effective intervention strategies to help these offenders and their families (Shorr, 1997; Dembo et al., 1999; Wasserman et al., 2000). Similar concerns are found within the educational and school psychology literature regarding the need for schools to better address mental health problems of children within our communities (McElhaney, Russell, & Barton, 1993; Koyanagi, 1999). With an estimated 70 percent of youngsters with mental health problems never receiving proper treatment (National Institute of Mental Health, 2001), there is a definite gap between needs and receipt of adequate treatment (Carlson, Tharinger, Bricklin, DeMers, & Paavola, 1996).

Research also shows that children who suffer one form of violence are prone to having experiences other types, such as community and family-related abuse and neglect (Saunders, 2003). Moreover, children who are treated for one form of trauma or psychopathology tend to have positive outcomes for other mental health problems simultaneously (Cohen, Mannarino, Murray, & Igelman, 2006). As such, there are very practical reasons to engage troubled youth, and when possible their families, as early as possible to enable these youngsters to develop prosocial coping mechanisms to deal with life issues.

Undoubtedly, the findings reported here raise some controversial public policy issues with regard to the prevention, intervention, and treatment of youngsters with serious forms of mental illness. Several key issues require consideration before making calls for broad changes in policy. For instance, what are the social and educational consequences of screening young children for mental disorders? Would such identification do more harm than good if it leads to further "labeling" troubled children in our schools? Do policies that target at-risk youths risk reinforcing negative stigmas or stereotypes so that children may come to believe they were "born" to be bad kids? Can we ethically force children to take treatment or do we "give up" on them if they or their families refuse? Moreover, who should pay for these interventions and screening processes if they are implemented? What is the unseen cost to society of *not* moving toward the early identification of mental problems in youth?

It is beyond the narrow scope of the present paper to offer definitive answers to each of these questions. In looking at these issues as a whole, however, the preliminary findings here support a larger body of literature that has suggested "interventions that reduce risk factors, while enhancing protective factors in family, school, peers, and community environments over the course of infant, child, and adolescent development hold promise for preventing multiple adolescent health and behavior problems (Catalano et al., 1988, p. 249). Many researchers in this area have encouraged the use of schools as ideal sites for the delivery of positive youth development programming (Bond & Compas, 1989; Durlak, 1995; Heide, 1999), behavioral monitoring (Bry, 1982), multidisciplinary mental health teams and school reorganization techniques (Cauce, Comer, & Schwartz, 1987; Comer, 1988), and the implementation of structured activities (Catalano et al., 1998) to reduce antisocial behaviors and improve academic and social competence in children. These programs would serve to complement needed interventions to reduce emotional and behavioral problems in juveniles within the criminal justice system, as well (Cohen et al., 1990; Dembo et al., 1999; MacKinnon-Lewis, Kaufman, & Frabutt, 2002). As exemplified within the present study, DSM-Oriented scales offer researchers another tool to help recognize mental health problems that may exist in these youths, especially if these children fall within borderline ranges that would be ignored with clinical diagnoses according to the DSM.

For such programs to be truly successful, however, better communication and cooperation is needed between schools, families, and various governmental agents throughout our communities to ensure that the mental health resources are available. The development of community-based committees, with representation from school administrators, teachers, parents, youths, criminal justice personnel and government officials, and academics, might offer some important first steps in fostering strong community ties to ensure the success of these programs. Complex issues will need to be tackled here such as: the availability of mental health programs, teacher training and sensitivity in dealing with emotionally-disorder youths, the cost effectiveness of testing for mental health problems, fostering parent cooperation and encouraging positive parenting techniques, and minimizing any potential stigmatization for youngsters who meet borderline or clinical levels of dysfunction. These issues are not easily reconciled and will require significant effort, money, and time before positive results might be seen. Recent research has suggested that multifocused intervention techniques that address mental health problems early in life have the best chance of meeting the needs of at-risk youth (Connor et al., 2007).

In a time when the public looks for easy solutions to social problems, the political ramifications of these types of policies may be a tough sell for public figures who look for quick results to get voters to the polls. The development of effective public information campaigns to reinforce community support will be essential if community-based approaches such as these are to become accepted and well established. Finally, objective assessments of "success" will require critical evaluations of program outcomes for youths and their families. Such programs must maintain flexibility to address the changing needs of families and offer greater sensitivity to gender, race, and cultural issues across communities.

Limitations and Future Research Directions

Not withstanding its many contributions, there are also some limitations to this study. These limitations include: 1) a largely atheoretical design, 2) the potential tautology of using DSM measures, and 3) the use of dichotomous variables. First, this study was largely atheoretical in that did not test specific theoretical hypotheses and assumptions. Instead, it operated within a general framework of mental health and developmental theory. Future research needs to pursue more theoretically-grounded research and consider how child and adolescent psychopathology may impact long-term offending throughout adulthood within specific lifecourse frameworks (e.g., Kempf, 1988; Moffitt, 1993; Tracy & Kempf-Leonard, 1996; Kempf-Leonard et al., 2001).

Secondly, the measures used here were based on DSM-oriented scales, which in turn are borrowed from emotional and behavioral symptoms within DSM diagnoses (American Psychiatric Association, 2000). Some critics have argued that there is an inherent tautology in using such behavioral indicators to first predict psychopathology and then to predict criminal or antisocial behaviors (Lahey & Waldman, 2005). In a recent attempt to address these concerns, some researchers have suggested distinguishing between synonymous items of temperament, conduct problems, and mental health measures to minimize the overlap across these measures. This "purification" of instruments measuring child and adolescent temperament typically involves excluding items such as those related to mental health or conduct disorders in the DSM and may be an important exercise in determining the unique value of such forms of psychopathology (Lemery, Essex, & Smider, 2002; Lahey & Waldman, 2005). When using these DSM-oriented scales in the future, researchers may want to consider excluding such items to determine if the predictive ability of these constructs remains without including such measures.

The present study design was sensitive to these concerns regarding tautological issues when dealing with studies involving behavioral measures. For instance, despite the fact that conduct disorder (CD) was a viable DSM-Oriented construct available within the Achenbach literature for replication, it was excluded here because of the inclusion of delinquent behaviors within the diagnostic criteria for CD. As the study was concerned with the prediction of serious offending behaviors, the use of delinquent CD behavioral indicators was potentially circular and purposefully avoided.

In contrast, the decision was made to use DSM-Oriented constructs for Affective Problems, ADHP, and ODP to avoid potential confounding or tautological issues in predicting serious offending. Most clinicians would agree that the criteria making up these diagnoses consist of non-criminal criteria. For example, Affective Problems included measures about mood, disposition, and feelings (e.g., enjoys little, cries, feels guilty, talks suicide, lacks energy, sad, etc.) that are neither criminal nor delinquent in orientation. ADHP included similar measures that captured information about a youth's failure to pay attention or impulsivity that are largely harmless to anyone but that child (e.g., fails to finish, doesn't cooperate, inattentive, talks too much, loud, etc.).   Lastly, ODP included measures regarding mood and temperament that in and of themselves do not constitute criminal actions, including arguing and acting defiant, stubbornness, or having a temper.   Moreover, the design included measures of previous acts of Serious Theft and Violence to control for earlier criminal acts that might contribute to the offending within that age block.

Another limitation here involves the decision to include dichotomized dependent variables for Serious Theft and Serious Violence. Some scholars have questioned the use of dichotomous variables versus categorical measures. These critics have cited the loss of potentially valuable information when measures are collapsed and concerns that dichotomization may lead to lower correlations between variables (Mertler & Vannatta, 2005). The advantages of using these dichotomous dependent variables are argued here to outweigh the limitations of dichotomization, because many of the independent and dependent variables of interest have nonlinear relationships (Loeber et al., 1998).   Additionally, the use of these dichotomous dependent variables, which were created by PYS staff, allows for both present and future comparisons with other PYS works that might employ similar measures. Although this study used dichotomous variables, an alternative would be to test categorical variables related to Serious Theft and Serious Violence and compare these results to see if the significant effects remain.

Lastly, the present study was restricted by the small number of childhood and adolescent DSM-Oriented mental health problems available for replication here. Moreover, as these measures are based largely upon the DSM and the behavioral indicators included there, this study did not take into account other cognitive or biological factors that have been shown in the empirical literature to have links with violence. The replication of the DSM-Oriented constructs also did not allow for the inclusion of measures of juvenile psychopathy, co-occurring alcohol and substance abuse, or the comorbidity of various mental health problems. Each of these issues is relevant to discussions on the etiology of violence and is commonly found within multi-problem youths entering the criminal justice system (Loeber et al., 1998; Dembo et al., 1999; Heide, 2004). Finally, gender differences also were unable to be addressed here due to the exclusion of girls within the PYS design.

With regard to future research, the present study utilized an exploratory approach by using logistic regression analyses to determine if bivariate and multivariate relationships were observed between mental health problems and types of offending behaviors. The present analyses highlighted the main effects of the models and did not take into account possible interaction effects between the variables. Certainly, the interesting findings that emerged here point toward the necessity for future research to pursue more complex statistical methods of analysis, such as employing latent growth curve, structural equation modeling, or pooled time series models. These more advanced statistical techniques offer the promise of yielding valuable information about the underlying causal mechanisms of mental health problems as they relate to violent behaviors, while potentially creating a more parsimonious model. An alternate statistical method worth consideration is Generalized Estimating Equation (GEE), which takes into account within-group differences. This population averaging method has been used to analyze longitudinal or clustered measurements similar to those found here (Hardin & Hilbe, 2003).

A different post-hoc method that is rarely employed involves a comparison of coefficients between models to determine whether significant differences might exist there (see Clogg, Petkova, & Haritou, 1995; Brame, Paternoster, Mazerolle, & Piquero, 1998; Allison, 1999). Also, to determine the effects of mental health problems with regard to within-group differences, further distinctions between types of violent offenders (e.g., homicide offenders versus all other violent offenders) could be made by conducting a rare events logistic regression (see King & Zeng, 2001; Piquero, MacDonald, Dobrin, Daigle, & Cullen, 2005). Such analyses could be a very important step in identifying the differing pathways that lead to violence.

In addition, a replication of this study using the youngest and oldest PYS samples would allow for a meaningful assessment of the significant mental health problems between these groups to see if these effects are replicated or change across the developmental periods. As this study began in the late 1980s and coincided with the peak of violent juvenile offending in the mid 1990s, it would be fascinating to see what DSM-oriented scales are significant predictors of serious offending within the older sample of the PYS, who had higher rates of serious offending. A comparison of T scores between these samples and with national means would also be quite useful to contrast Pittsburgh these cohorts. Similarly, a study replication using data from the two other sites involved in the original Causes and Correlates of Delinquency studies (Denver and Rochester) would allow for a determination of whether these results are limited to this region or if they are able more generalizable to other geographical locations around the country. Another meaningful investigation might be to conduct a follow up with the approximate 17 percent of PYS participants and their families who have dropped out of the study through attrition. Through the use of adult criminal record checks and follow-up interviews, it would be useful to compare the outcomes for these subjects versus those found here. This would be an important exercise as "studies have shown that attrition usually is not random, but takes a disproportionate toll on those participants who are most at risk and most essential to the topic of investigation" (Loeber et al., 1998, p. 18). These suggestions for future research are an important next step in the quest to identify what role mental health factors have in the temporal development of serious offending behaviors over the lifecourse.

Concluding Remarks

In conclusion, this study has presented a number of important findings with regard to the "reach" of mental health problems, such as Affective, Attention-Deficit/Hyperactivity, and Oppositional Defiant Problems, in predicting Serious Theft and Serious Violence in youngsters. This topic is particularly relevant today in light of public concerns about juvenile crime and the increasing number of youngsters entering our criminal justice system with co-occurring mental disorders. While working within a developmental and lifecourse orientation, this research utilized an innovative form of measurement, or DSM-oriented scales, to further explore how forms of childhood and adolescent psychopathology may influence poor life outcomes.

A multitude of studies have identified three key effects that are salient to understanding violence: age, time (period), and cohort effects. Each of these elements is fundamental in identifying the "temporal trends of health in general and of violence trends in particular". (Fabio et al., 2006, p. 152). The present study is an attempt to address these complexities. Using longitudinal, multiple-respondent, and multiple-instrument data collection, the findings here point to some of the possible relationships that may explain later violence in the lifecourse.

Thus, this work offers a considerable contribution toward the understanding of what role mental illness may play in the development of serious offending. Despite recent advances in criminology and psychology to understand serious juvenile offending, there is certainly much more research to be done to uncover the diverse origins of interpersonal violence (Reiss & Roth, 1993), especially with regard to the role that psychological dysfunction may play early in the lifecourse (Loeber et al.,

1998; Loeber, 2004). Toward this end, this work has offered numerous substantive, methodological, and policy suggestions that will propel scientists toward the answers to many of the important questions raised here. It is our hope that this study will encourage others to ponder and investigate these complex mechanisms even further, united with the ultimate goal of creating future generations of healthy families and children within our communities.

Appendix A: Reliability of DSM-Oriented Constructs

	ODP-P	ADHP-P	ANX-P	AFF-P	ODP-T	ADHP-T	ANX-T	AFF-T
PHASE A								
ALPHA	.7403	.7992	.5693	.5940	.8806	.9246	.6660	.7003
n	492	499	499	499	453	443	396	425
PHASE B								
ALPHA	.7097	.7823	.5457	.5250	.8982	.9413	.5713	.6878
n	483	484	483	382	462	442	412	444
PHASE C								
ALPHA	.7329	.8002	.5512	.5637	.9027	.9404	.6285	.6863
n	468	467	468	467	449	431	398	418
PHASE D								
ALPHA	.7917	.8085	.5766	.6240	.9193	.9465	.5467	.6871
n	474	475	475	474	433	420	384	402
PHASE E								
ALPHA	.7312	.8211	.5627	.5892	.9124	.9447	.6724	.6925
n	478	476	478	477	424	421	375	399
PHASE F								
ALPHA	.7643	.8303	.5813	.5717	.9156	.9482	.6358	.7356
n	481	481	481	481	446	436	395	416

Continued on next page

Appendix A continued

PHASE G	ODP-P	ADHP-P	ANX-P	AFF-P	ODP-T	ADHP-T	ANX-T	AFF-T
ALPHA	.7980	.8276	.5829	.6305	.9142	.9493	.6854	7479
n	465	465	464	465	432	426	379	403
PHASE H	ODP-P	ADHP-P	ANX-P	AFF-P	ODP-T	ADHP-T	ANX-T	AFF-T
ALPHA	.7667	.8238	.5366	.6003	.9133	.9485	.7169	.7296
n	465	464	464	463	418	411	382	396
PHASE J	ODP-P	ADHP-P	ANX-P	AFF-P	ODP-T	ADHP-T	ANX-T	AFF-T
ALPHA	.7764	.8233	.5875	.6345	.9038	.9513	.6986	.7225
n	469	469	469	469	431	424	372	393
PHASE L	ODP-P	ADHP-P	ANX-P	AFF-P	ODP-T	ADHP-T	ANX-T	AFF-T
ALPHA	.7918	.8279	.5608	.6233	.9105	.9543	.7010	.7406
n	463	463	462	463	432	426	380	399
PHASE N	ODP-P	ADHP-P	ANX-P	AFF-P	ODP-T	ADHP-T	ANX-T	AFF-T
ALPHA	.7813	.8419	.6026	.5982	.9195	.9537	.6836	.7563
n	454	455	456	454	424	412	373	386
PHASE P	ODP-P	ADHP-P	ANX-P	AFF-P	ODP-T	ADHP-T	ANX-T	AFF-T
ALPHA	.8224	.8274	.6036	.6151	.9094	.9483	.6268	.7351
n	440	440	440	440	381	371	306	314

Continued on next page

Appendix A continued

PHASE R	ODP-P	ADHP-P	ANX-P	AFF-P	ODP-T	ADHP-T	ANX-T	AFF-T
ALPHA	.7952	.8263	.6129	.7440	.9117	.9448	MISSING	MISSING
n	427	435	435	435	315	292	MISSING	MISSING

PHASE T	ODP-P	ADHP-P	ANX-P	AFF-P	ODP-T	ADHP-T	ANX-T	AFF-T
ALPHA	.7746	.7909	.6666	.7292	N/A	N/A	N/A	N/A
n	411	434	411	434	N/A	N/A	N/A	N/A

Appendix B: CBCL DSM-Oriented Scales Raw Scores, T Scores,
              and Items

Oppositional Defiant Problems

Age 6-11		Age 12-18		Items
Raw	T	Raw	T	
0	50	0	50	3. Argues
1	51	1	51	22. Disobedient at home
2	52	2	52	23. Disobedient at school
3	55	3	55	86. Stubborn
4	58	4	58	95. Temper
5	62	5	62	
6	66	6	66	5 items total
7	70	7	69	
8	73	8	71	
9	77	9	75	
10	80	10	80	

No data missing when converted from 1991 to 2001

Attention Deficit/Hyperactivity

Age 6-11		Age 12-18		Items
Raw	T	Raw	T	
0-2	50	0-1	50	4. Fails to finish
3	51	2	51	8. Can't cooperate
4	53	3	52	10. Can't sit still
5	56	4	55	41. Impulsive
6	58	5	57	78. Inattentive
7	60	6	59	93. Talks too much
8	62	7	62	104. Loud
9	66	8	65	

Continued on next page

Appendix B continued

Age 6-11		Age 12-18		
Raw	*T*	*Raw*	*T*	
10	69	9	67	7 items total
11	72	10	68	
12	75	11	70	
13	77	12	73	
14	80	13	77	
		14	80	

No data missing when converted from 1991 to 2001

Anxiety Problems

Age 6-11		Age 12-18		*Items*
Raw	*T*	*Raw*	*T*	
0	50	0	50	11. Dependent
1	51	1	53	29. Fears things other than school
2	55	2	58	30. Fears school
3	60	3	62	45. Nervous
4	65	4	66	50. Fearful
5	68	5	70	112. Worries
6	70	6	71	
7	72	7	73	6 items total
8	73	8	74	
9	75	9	76	
10	77	10	77	
11	78	11	79	
12	80	12	80	

No data missing when converted from 1991 to 2001

Continued on next page

Appendix B continued

Affective Problems

Age 6-11		Age 12-18		
Raw	T	Raw	T	*Items*
0	50	0	50	5. Enjoys little
1	52	1	52	14. Cries
2	56	2	55	18. Harms self
3	60	3	59	24. Doesn't eat well
4	63	4	61	35. Feels worthless
5	65	5	63	52. Feels too guilty
6	68	6	66	54. Tired
7	70	7	67	76. Sleeps less than others
8	72	8	70	77. Sleeps more than others
9	73	9	72	91. Talks suicide
10	75	10	73	100. Sleep problems
11	76	11	75	102. Lacks energy
12	78	12	77	103. Sad
13	79	13	78	
14	81	14	80	13 items total
15	83	15	82	
16	84	16	83	
17	86	17	85	
18	87	18	87	
19	89	19	88	
20	91	20	90	

Continued on next page

Appendix B continued

Affective Problems

Age 6-11		Age 12-18		Items
Raw	T	Raw	T	
21	92	21	92	
22	94	22	93	
23	95	23	95	
24	97	24	97	
25	98	25	98	
26	100	26	100	
Item #5 missing data				

Appendix C: TRF DSM-Oriented Scales Raw Scores, T Scores,
                       and Items

Oppositional Defiant Problems

Age 6-11		Age 12-18		*Items*
Raw	*T*	*Raw*	*T*	
0	50	0	50	3. Argues
1	54	1	54	6. Defiant
2	58	2	58	23. Disobedient at school
3	60	3	61	86. Stubborn
4	62	4	63	95. Temper
5	63	5	65	
6	66	6	66	5 items total
7	68	7	69	
8	70	8	70	
9	72	9	72	
10	75	10	75	

No data missing when converted from 1991 to 2001
No data available at Phase T

Attention Deficit/Hyperactivity

Age 6-11		Age 12-18		*Items*
Raw	*T*	*Raw*	*T*	
0-3	50	0-2	50	4. Fails to finish
4	51	3	51	8. Can't concentrate
5	52	4	52	10. Can't sit still
6	53	5	53	15. Fidgets
7	54	6	54	22. Doesn't follow directions
8	55	7	55	24. Disturbs others
9	56	8	56	41. Impulsive
10	57	9	57	53. Talks out
11	58	10	58	67. Disrupts

Continued on next page

Appendix C continued

Age 6-11		Age 12-18		
Raw	*T*	*Raw*	*T*	
12	59	11	59	78. Inattentive
13	60	12	60	93. Talks much
				100. Doesn't complete
14	61	13	61	tasks
15	62	14	62	104. Loud
16	63	15	63	
17	64	16	64	13 items total
18	65	17	65	
19	66	18	66	
20	67	19	67	
21	68	20	68	
22	70	21	69	
23	73	22	70	
24	75	23	73	
25	78	24	75	
26	80	25	78	
		26	80	

No data missing when converted from 1991 to 2001
No data available at Phase T

Anxiety Problems

Age 6-11		Age 12-18		*Items*
Raw	*T*	*Raw*	*T*	
0	50	0	50	11. Dependent
				29. Fears things other
1	56	1	56	school
2	61	2	62	30. Fears school
3	65	3	65	45. Nervous
4	68	4	68	50. Fearful
5	70	5	70	112. Worries

Continued on next page

Appendix C continued

Age 6-11		Age 12-18		
Raw	*T*	*Raw*	*T*	
6	71	6	71	6 items total
7	73	7	73	
8	74	8	74	
9	76	9	76	
10	77	10	77	
11	79	11	79	
12	80	12	80	

No data missing when converted from 1991 to 2001
No data available Phase R & T

Affective Problems

Age 6-11		Age 12-18		Items
Raw	*T*	*Raw*	*T*	
0	50	0	50	5. Enjoys little
1	54	1	52	14. Cries
2	57	2	55	18. Harms self
3	60	3	58	35. Feels worthless
4	63	4	61	52. Feels too guilty
5	65	5	62	54. Tired
6	67	6	64	60. Apathetic
7	69	7	67	91. Talks suicide
8	70	8	69	102. Lacks energy
9	73	9	70	103. Sad
10	75	10	73	
11	78	11	75	10 items total
12	80	12	78	
13	83	13	81	
14	85	14	84	
15	88	15	86	

Continued on next page

Appendix C continued

Age 6-11		Age 12-18	
Raw	T	Raw	T
16	90	16	89
17	93	17	92
18	95	18	95
19	98	19	97
20	100	20	100

Item #5 missing data
No data available at Phase R
No data available at Phase T

Appendix D: Summary Univariate Statistics

Independent Variables	N	Mean	SD	Normal Range (%)	Borderline range (%)	Clinical T score range (%)	Borderline + Clinical (%)
Oppositional Defiant Age Blk 1 (P)	502	56.64	5.28	92.8	4.0	2.2	6.2
Oppositional Defiant Age Blk 2 (P)	483	56.40	5.66	89.9	7.2	2.9	10.1
Oppositional Defiant Age Blk 3 (P)	471	55.90	5.63	91.9	4.9	3.2	8.1
Attention Deficit Age Blk 1 (P)	502	54.85	4.99	94.0	5.2	0.8	6.0
Attention Deficit Age Blk 2 (P)	483	54.45	5.24	94.8	3.8	1.4	5.2
Attention Deficit Age Blk 3 (P)	471	54.01	4.94	95.5	3.0	1.5	4.5
Anxiety Age Blk 1 (P)	502	53.36	4.16	97.0	2.4	0.6	3.0
Anxiety Age Blk 2 (P)	483	52.82	3.86	98.3	1.3	0.4	1.7
Anxiety Age Blk 3 (P)	471	52.92	4.08	97.2	2.4	0.4	2.8
Affective Age Blk 1 (P)	502	54.12	4.29	98.0	1.6	0.4	2.0
Affective Age Blk 2 (P)	483	52.82	3.72	99.0	0.8	0.2	1.0
Affective Age Blk 3 (P)	471	53.02	3.95	98.3	1.3	0.4	1.7
Oppositional Defiant Age Blk 1 (T)	502	57.51	6.32	84.3	13.1	2.6	15.7
Oppositional Defiant Age Blk 2 (T)	485	58.94	6.86	77.9	15.5	6.6	22.1
Oppositional Defiant Age Blk 3 (T)	463	58.56	6.92	77.1	14.7	8.2	22.9
Attention Deficit Age Blk 1 (T)	502	57.18	6.11	85.9	11.3	2.8	14.1
Attention Deficit Age Blk 2 (T)	484	58.46	7.05	80.0	13.2	6.8	20.0
Attention Deficit Age Blk 3 (T)	463	58.60	6.96	79.7	11.4	8.9	20.3
Anxiety Age Blk 1 (T)	502	54.49	4.45	96.2	3.6	0.2	3.8
Anxiety Age Blk 2 (T)	483	55.04	4.93	94.2	5.0	0.8	5.8

Continued on next page

Appendix D continued

Independent Variables	N	Mean	SD	Normal Range (%)	Borderline range (%)	Clinical T score range (%)	Borderline + Clinical (%)
Anxiety Age Blk 3 (T)	458	54.71	5.61	91.5	6.8	1.7	8.5
Affective Age Blk 1 (T)	502	55.31	4.18	97.6	2.2	0.2	2.4
Affective Age Blk 2 (T)	483	56.13	4.67	95.2	3.8	1.0	4.8
Affective Age Blk 3 (T)	459	55.75	5.23	93.7	4.8	1.5	6.3
Dependent Variables	*N*	*Mean*	*SD*				
Serious Theft Age Blk 2	485	.08	.27				
Serious Theft Age Blk 3	475	.16	.37				
Serious Theft Age Blk 4	452	.07	.25				
Serious Violence Age Blk 2	485	.10	.30				
Serious Violence Age Blk 3	477	.21	.41				
Serious Violence Age Blk 4	453	.08	.28				
Control Variables	*N*	*Mean*	*SD*				
Family SES Age Blk 1	502	1.98	.68				
Family SES Age Blk 2	485	1.98	.68				
Family SES Age Blk 3	474	2.01	.70				
Race	503	1.58	.49				
Physical Aggression	502	.26	.44				

Note. Blk 1 = Age blocked data for middle childhood or approximate ages 7 to 9 years old. Blk 2 = Age blocked data or late childhood or approximate ages 10 to 12 years old. Blk 3 = Age blocked data for early adolescence or approximate ages 13 to 16 years old. Blk 4 = Age blocked data for late adolescence or approximate ages 17 to 19 years old. SES = socioeconomic status.

Appendix E: Zero-Order Pearson Correlations of Independent, Dependent, and Control Variables in Full Model

	1	2	3	4	5	6	7	8	9	10
1. Family SES Chunk 1										
2. Family SES Chunk 2	.610*									
3. Family SES Chunk 3	.420*	.510*								
4. Race	.117*	.090*	.087							
5. Physical Agg Chunk 1	-.034	-.045	-.058	.075						
6. ODP (P) Chunk 1	-.006	.019	-.029	-.067	.188*					

Continued on next page

Appendix E continued

	1	2	3	4	5	6	7	8	9	10
7. ODP (P) Chunk 2	-.006	-.014	-.076	-.015	.167*	.770*				
8. ODP (P) Chunk 3	.006	.002	-.084	-.034	.149*	.612*	.750*			
9. ADHP (P) Chunk 1	-.002	-.023	.026	.080	.149*	.701*	.596*	.503*		
10. ADHP (P) Chunk 2	-.020	-.056	-.061	.053	.161*	.589*	.726*	.591*	.778*	
11. ADHP (P) Chunk 3	-.003	-.011	-.033	.045	.121*	.500*	.613*	.740*	.652*	.789*

Continued on next page

Appendix E continued

	1	2	3	4	5	6	7	8	9	10
12. Anx Prob (P) Chunk 1	-.066	-.064	-.030	-.059	.052	.446*	.365*	.263*	.524*	.440*
13. Anx Prob (P) Ck 2	-.069	-.088	-.093	-.027	.018	.289*	.418*	.315*	.360*	.519*
14. Anx Prob (P) Ck 3	-.014	-.022	-.072	-.008	.051	.284*	.379*	.415*	.363*	.454*
15. Aff Prob (P) Ck 1	-.053	-.011	.006	-.092	.086	.508*	.412*	.296*	.521*	.423*
16. Aff Prob (P) C 2	-.046	-.083	-.083	-.101*	.031	.388*	.549*	.381*	.372*	.516*
17. Aft Prob (P) Chunk 3	.012	-.025	-.132*	-.090	.088	.276*	.400*	.479*	.293*	.394*

Continued on next page

Appendix E continued

	1	2	3	4	5	6	7	8	9	10
18. ODP (T) Chunk 1	.122*	.147*	.141*	.342*	.180*	.342*	.331*	.257*	.357*	.308*
19. ODP (T) Chunk 2	.141*	.182*	.185*	.343*	.154*	.312*	.345*	.277*	.335*	.345*
20. ODP (T) Chunk 3	.208*	.228*	.213*	.323*	.175*	.250*	.311*	.343*	.260*	.275*
21. ADHP (T) Chunk 1	.088*	.112*	.117*	.275*	.106*	.334*	.314*	.234*	.428*	.383*
22. ADHP (T) Chunk 2	.135*	.153*	.200*	.279*	.144*	.280*	.274*	.243*	.344*	.357*

Continued on next page

Appendix E continued

	1	2	3	4	5	6	7	8	9	10
23. ADHP (T) Chunk 3	.221*	.185*	.218*	.325*	.153*	.240*	.285*	.342*	.281*	.294*
24. Anxiety Prob (T) Chunk 1	-.015	-.031	-.040	-.038	.009	.249*	.164*	.161*	.404*	.323*
25. Anxiety Prob (T) Chunk 2	.024	.076	.028	-.024	.028	.195*	.183*	.169*	.300*	.256*
26. Anxiety Prob (T) Chunk 3	.117*	.130*	.109*	.036	.140*	.179*	.186*	.180*	.251*	.262*

Continued on next page

Appendix E continued

	1	2	3	4	5	6	7	8	9	10
27. Affect Prob (T) Chunk 1	.148*	.146*	.124*	.248*	.044	.220*	.221*	.134*	.334*	.295*
28. Affect Prob (T) Chunk 2	.127*	.149*	.126*	.176*	.090*	.210*	.230*	.176*	.306*	.290*
29. Affect Prob (T) Chunk 3	.166*	.184*	.130*	.172*	.110*	.094*	.142*	.196*	.131*	.129*
30. Serious Theft Chunk 2	.077	.020	.018	.071	.054	.058	.06	.001	.100*	.104*
31. Serious Theft Chunk 3	.121*	.147*	.085	.036	.006	.047	.080	.109*	.039	.053

Continued on next page

Appendix E continued

	1	2	3	4	5	6	7	8	9	10
32. Serious Theft Chunk 4	.018	.085	.026	-.106*	-.014	.036	.041	.058	-.024	.004
33. Serious Viol Chunk 2	.022	.070	.045	.151*	.182*	.096*	.113*	.039	.123*	.127*
34. Serious Viol Chunk 3	.107*	.138*	.115*	.167*	.061	.108*	.143*	.153*	.099*	.118*
35. Serious Viol Chunk 4	.041	.030	.000	.105*	.022	.073	.148*	.137*	.079	.126*

Continued on next page

Continued on next page

Appendix E continued

	11	12	13	14	15	16	17	18	19	20
12. Anx Prob (P) Chunk 1	.368*									
13. Anx Prob (P) Ck 2	.432*	.654*								
14. Anx Prob (P) Ck 3	.566*	.505*	.653*							
15. Aff Prob (P) Ck 1	.315*	.623*	.431*	.368*						
16. Aff Prob (P) C k2	.390*	.444*	.581*	.457*	.634*					
17. Aff Prob (P) Chunk 3	.508*	.340*	.418*	.649*	.389*	.544*				

Continued on next page

Appendix E continued

	11	12	13	14	15	16	17	18	19	20
18. ODP (T) Chunk 1	.318*	.138*	.124*	.180*	.072	.087	.111*			
19. ODP (T) Chunk 2	.362*	.131*	.108*	.153*	.077	.109*	.065	.739*		
20. ODP (T) Chunk 3	.349*	.064	.129*	.142*	.089	.126*	.144*	.550*	.638*	
21. ADHP (T) Chunk 1	.368*	.158*	.113*	.137*	.067	.083	.053	.836*	.667*	.487*
22. ADHP (T) Chunk 2	.379*	.138*	.113*	.135*	.048	.079	.045	.635*	.861*	.577*

Continued on next page

Appendix E continued

	11	12	13	14	15	16	17	18	19	20
23. ADHP (T) Chunk 3	.379*	.053	.132*	.155*	.073	.094*	.118*	.469*	.569*	.844*
24. Anx Prob (T) Chunk 1	.303*	.315*	.255*	.191*	.189*	.146*	.097*	.399*	.298*	.154*
25. Anx Prob (T) Chunk 2	.278*	.231*	.232*	.178*	.094*	.135*	.088	.381*	.451*	.272*
26. Anx Prob (T) Ck 3	.276*	.155*	.236*	.219*	.143*	.159*	.140*	.340*	.351*	.462*
27. Aff Prob (T) Chunk 1	.251*	.158*	.158*	.140*	.143*	.182*	.143*	.548*	.438*	.365*
28. Aff Prob (T) Chunk 2	.287*	.185*	.204*	.155*	.111	.162*	.143*	.433*	.605*	.375*

Continued on next page

Appendix E continued

	11	12	13	14	15	16	17	18	19	20
29. Aff Prob (T) Chunk 3	.198*	.080	.147*	.170*	.099*	.136*	.173*	.274*	.298*	.509*
30. Serious Theft Chunk 2	.081	-.006	.036	.046	.000	.035	.038	.169*	.161*	.222*
31. Serious Theft Chunk 3	.179*	-.019	-.030	.027	.017	-.004	.050	.211*	.276*	.330*
32. Serious Theft Chunk 4	.037	-.044	-.010	-.015	-.070	-.031	.054	-.025	.059	.104*
33. Serious Viol Chunk 2	.139*	.081	.066	.098	.099*	.077	.097*	.221*	.241*	.193*

Continued on next page

Appendix E continued

	11	12	13	14	15	16	17	18	19	20
34. Serious Viol Chunk 3	.165*	.028	.051	.146*	.092*	.116*	.148*	.329*	.352*	.381*
35. Serious Viol Chunk 4	.114*	-.042	.021	.106*	.018	.086	.082	.137*	.227*	.253*

Continued on next page

Appendix E continued

	21	22	23	24	25	26	27	28	29	30
22. ADHP (T) Chunk 2	.698*									
23. ADHP (T) Chunk 3	.482*	.584*								
24. Anx Prob (T) Chunk 1	.484*	.319*	.139*							
25. Anx Prob (T) Chunk 2	.350*	.523*	.259*	.468*						
26. Anx Prob (T) Chunk 3	.592*	.354*	.452*	.288*	.407*					

Continued on next page

Appendix E continued

	21	22	23	24	25	26	27	28	29	30
27. Aff Prob (T) Chunk 1	.477*	.440*	.353*	.507*	.343*	.301*				
28. Aff Prob (T) Chunk 2	.273*	.617*	.344*	.355*	.555*	.302*	.553*			
29. Aff Prob (T) Chunk 3	.273*	.298*	.472*	.038*	.148*	.504*	.202*	.346*		
30. Serious Theft Chunk 2	.142*	.160*	.183*	.023	.097*	.122*	.156*	.120*	.142*	
31. Serious Theft Chunk 3	.179*	.280*	.281*	.064	.113*	.175*	.158*	.210*	.190*	.372*
32. Ser Theft Chunk 4	-.024	.051	.102*	-.028	.049	.035*	.016	.091	-.021	.121*

Continued on next page

Appendix E continued

	21	22	23	24	25	26	27	28	29	30
33. Serious Viol Chunk 2	.177*	.198*	.155*	.054	.030	.172*	.202*	.155*	.185*	.278*
34. Serious Viol Chunk 3	.295*	.355*	.325*	.081	.165*	.197*	.282*	265*	.238*	.291*
35. Serious Viol Chunk 4	.077	.203*	.195*	-.044	.069	.065	.060	.149*	.104*	.159*
	31	32	33	34	35					
32. Serious Theft Chunk 4	.347									
33. Ser Viol Chunk 2	.247*	.061								

Continued on next page

Appendix E continued

	21	22	23	24	25	26	27	28	29	30
34. Serious Viol Chunk 3	.410*	.126*	.323*							
35. Serious Viol Chunk 4	.275*	.212*	.092	.293*						

Note. ODP = Oppositional Defiant Problems. ADHP = Attention Deficit/Hyperactivity Problems. Anxiety Prob = Anxiety Problems. Affect Prob = Affective Problems. Physical Agg = Physical aggression. (P) = Parent instrument. (T) = Teacher instrument. SES = socioeconomic status.

$p < .05$.

Appendix F: Logistic Regression Models 1-3: Effects of Parent Reports of DSM-Oriented Problems at Age Block 1 on Serious Theft Behaviors at Age Blocks 2, 3, and 4

Independent Variables:	MODEL 1: AGE BLOCK 2 on 1					MODEL 2: AGE BLOCK 3 on 1				
	b	se(b)	OR	Lower 95% CL	Upper 95% CL	b	se(b)	OR	Lower 95% CL	Upper 95% CL
Oppositional Defiant Problems	.003	.045	1.003	.919	1.096	.026	.039	1.026	.951	1.107
Attention Deficit/Hyperactivity Problems	.084	.046	1.087	.993	1.190	-.007	.042	.993	.913	1.079
Anxiety Problems	-.046	.059	.955	.852	1.072	-.036	.049	.965	.876	1.063
Affective Problems	-.030	.055	.970	.872	1.080	.014	.044	1.014	.930	1.105
Control Variables:										
Serious Theft (Age Block 2)	--	--	--	--	--	2.262*	.402	9.600	4.370	21.088
Serious Theft (Age Block 3)	--	--	--	--	--	--	--	--	--	--
Physical Aggression	.260	.375	1.296	.621	2.705	-.269	.340	.764	.392	1.489
Serious Violence (Age Block 2)	--	--	--	--	--	1.193*	.387	3.297	1.543	7.046
Serious Violence (Age Bk 3)	--	--	--	--	--	--	--	--	--	--

Continued on next page

Appendix F continued

Independent Variables:	b	se(b)	OR	Lower 95% CL	Upper 95% CL	b	se(b)	OR	Lower 95% CL	Upper 95% CL
Family SES (Age Block 1):	.868	.565	2.383	.787	7.216	.319	.510	1.375	.506	3.740
Low	.722	.512	2.059	.756	5.612	.118	.437	1.125	.477	2.652
Typical										
Family SES (Age Block 2):	--	--	--	--	--	1.021*	.511	2.775	1.020	7.552
Low	--	--	--	--	--	.469	.447	1.598	.665	3.838
Typical										
Family SES (Age Block 3):						--	--	--	--	--
Low	--	--	--	--	--	--	--	--	--	--
Typical										
Race (Black)	.367	.375	1.296	.621	2.705	-.058	.296	.944	.528	1.687
Constant	-4.157					-2.606				
-2 Log Likelihood	259.489					355.616				

Continued on next page

Appendix F continued

Independent Variables:	b	se(b)	OR	Lower 95% CL	Upper 95% CL	b	se(b)	OR	Lower 95% CL	Upper 95% CL
% Correct Classification (Controls)	92.0					86.1				
% Correct Classification (Full Model)	92.0					86.1				
Model χ^2	11.893					68.281*				
Pseudo R^2 Controls only	.033					.224				
Pseudo R^2 Full model	.057					.227				
N	485					474				

(Continued on next page)

Appendix F continued

Independent Variables:	MODEL 3: AGE BLOCK 4 on 1				
	b	*se(b)*	*OR*	Lower 95% CL	Upper 95% CL
Oppositional Defiant Problems	.048	.060	1.050	.933	1.181
Attention Deficit/Hyperactivity Problems	-.040	.068	.961	.841	1.098
Anxiety Problems	.048	.073	1.049	.909	1.210
Affective Problems	-.142	.078	.867	.745	1.010
Control Variables:					
Serious Theft (Age Block 2)	-.118	.627	.888	.260	3.035
	2.672	.534	14.466	5.081	41.185
Serious Theft (Age Block 3)	.145	.522	1.156	.416	3.218
	-.089	.712	.915	.226	3.694
Physical Aggression Serious Violence (Age Block 2)	.263	.543	1.301	.449	3.773
Serious Violence (Age Block 3)					
Family SES (Age Block 1): Low	-.808	.877	.446	.080	2.489
	.446	.655	1.562	.433	5.637
	1.051	.844	2.860	.547	14.964
Typical	.313	.670	1.368	.368	5.090
Family SES (Age Block 2): Low	-.591	.761	.554	.125	2.461
	-.381	.599	.683	.211	2.210
Typical					
Family SES (Age Block 3): Low					
Typical					
Race (Black)	-1.182*	.472	.307	.122	.773

Continued on next page

Appendix F continued

Constant	1.242				
-2 Log Likelihood	163.375				
% Correct Classification (Controls)	93.4				
% Correct Classification (Full Model)	93.0				
Model χ^2	55.666*				
Pseudo R^2 Controls only	.279				
Pseudo R^2 Full model	.303				
N	440				

Note. CL = Confidence limit, 95% CL calculated as $\beta \pm$ (1.96 standard error). SES = socioeconomic status.
*$p < .05$.

Appendix G: Logistic Regression Models 4-5: Effects of Parent Reports of DSM-Oriented Problems at Age Block 2 on Serious Theft Behaviors at Age Blocks 3 and 4

Independent Variables:	MODEL 4: AGE BLOCK 2 on 3					MODEL 5: AGE BLOCK 2 on 4				
	b	se(b)	OR	Lower 95% CL	Upper 95% CL	b	se(b)	OR	Lower 95% CL	Upper 95% CL
Oppositional Defiant Problems	.052	.035	1.053	.983	1.129	.027	.055	1.027	.922	1.144
Attention Deficit/Hyperactivity Problems	.003	.041	1.003	.926	1.086	-.037	.064	.964	.850	1.093
Anxiety Problems	-.050	.049	.951	.864	1.047	.053	.071	1.055	.918	1.212
Affective Problems	-.026	.051	.974	.881	1.077	-.073	.080	.929	.794	1.088
Control Variables:										
Serious Theft (Age Block 2)	2.551*	.389	12.824	5.980	27.500	-.015	.611	.986	.298	3.265
Serious Theft (Age Block 3)	--	--	--	--	--	2.636*	.511	13.961	5.127	38.014
Physical Aggression										
Serious Violence (Age Block 2)										
Serious Violence (Age Block 3)										

Continued on next page

Appendix G continued

Independent Variables:	b	se(b)	OR	Lower 95% CL	Upper 95% CL	b	se(b)	OR	Lower 95% CL	Upper 95% CL
Family SES (Age Block 1):										
Low	.350	.511	1.420	.522	3.862	-.421	.901	.657	.112	3.840
	.172	.441	1.187	.500	2.817	.819	.716	2.268	.557	9.232
	1.068*	.504	2.909	1.083	7.820	1.024	.815	2.783	.564	13.740
Typical	.411	.444	1.508	.632	3.600	.095	.692	1.100	.283	4.267
Family SES (Age Block 2):										
Low	--	--	--	--	--	-.712	.751	.491	.113	2.137
	--	--	--	--	--	-.520	.607	.594	.181	1.954
Typical										
Family SES (Age Block 3):										
Low										
Typical										
Race (Black)	.057	.289	1.059	.601	1.866	-1.090*	.457	.336	.137	.823
Constant	-1.767					-1.794				
-2 Log Likelihood	355.963					164.321				

Continued on next page

Appendix G continued

% Correct Classification (Controls)	85.6		93.6		
% Correct Classification (Full Model)	85.4		936		
Model χ^2	63.96*		49.18*		
Pseudo R^2 Controls only	.201		.268		
Pseudo R^2 Full model	.215		.275		
N	472		438		

Note. CL = Confidence limit, 95% CL calculated as $\beta \pm$ (1.96 standard error). SES = socioeconomic status.
*$p < .05$.

Appendix H: Logistic Regression Model 6: Effects of Parent Reports of DSM-Oriented Problems at Age Block 3 on Serious Theft Behaviors at Age Block 4

Independent Variables:	*MODEL 6: AGE BLOCK 3 on 4*				
	b	*se(b)*	*OR*	Lower 95% CL	Upper 95% CL
Oppositional Defiant Problems	.028	.059	1.029	.916	1.155
Attention Deficit/Hyperactivity Problems	-.032	.071	.969	.842	1.114
Anxiety Problems	-.132	.099	.876	.722	1.063
Affective Problems	.086	.073	1.090	.944	1.259
Control Variables:					
Serious Theft (Age Block 2)	.122	.614	1.130	.339	3.767
Serious Theft (Age Block 3)	2.751*	.522	15.664	5.636	43.531
Physical Aggression Serious Violence (Age Block 2)					
Serious Violence (Age Block 3)					
Family SES (Age Block 1): Low	-.915	.872	.401	.073	2.211
	.695	.649	2.005	.562	7.148
	1.245	.805	3.474	.717	16.821
Typical	.007	.663	1.007	.274	3.694
Family SES (Age Block 2): Low	-.908	.797	.403	.085	1.926
	-.383	.609	.682	.207	2.247
Typical					
Family SES (Age Block 3): Low					
Typical					
					Continued on next page

Appendix H continued

Independent Variables:	b	se(b)	OR	Lower 95% CL	Upper 95% CL
Race (Black)	-1.255*	.486	.285	.110	.740
Constant		-.757			
-2 Log Likelihood		158.635			
% Correct Classification (Controls) % Correct Classification (Full Model)		93.6 93.8			
Model χ^2		54.87*			
Pseudo R^2 Controls only Pseudo R^2 Full model		.288 .305			
N		438			

Note. CL = Confidence limit, 95% CL calculated as $\beta \pm (1.96$ standard error). SES = socioeconomic status.
*$p < .05$.

Appendix I: Logistic Regression Models 7-9: Effects of Teacher Reports of DSM-Oriented Problems at Age Block 1 on Serious Theft Behaviors at Age Blocks 2, 3, and 4

	MODEL 7: AGE BLOCK 2 on 1					MODEL 8: AGE BLOCK 3 on 1				
Independent Variables:	b	se(b)	OR	Lower 95% CL	Upper 95% CL	b	se(b)	OR	Lower 95% CL	Upper 95% CL
Oppositional Defiant Problems	.073	.046	1.075	.982	1.178	.068	.040	1.071	.990	1.158
Attention Deficit/Hyperactivity Problems	.011	.049	1.011	.918	1.113	.007	.042	1.007	.927	1.093
Anxiety Problems	-.084	.049	.919	.835	1.012	-.017	.039	.983	.910	1.062
Affective Problems	.100*	.049	1.106	1.004	1.217	.014	.043	1.014	.932	1.104
Control Variables:										
Serious Theft (Age Block 2)	--	--	--	--	--	2.125*	.404	8.371	3.792	18.478
Serious Theft (Age Block 3)	--	--	--	--	--	--	--	--	--	--
Physical Aggression	.153	.381	1.165	.552	2.460	-.397	.343	.672	.343	1.316
Serious Violence (Age Block 2)	--	--	--	--	--	1.035*	.386	2.817	1.320	6.007
Serious Violence (Age Block 3)	--	--	--	--	--	--	--	--	--	--

Continued on next page

Appendix I continued

Independent Variables:	b	se(b)	OR	Lower 95% CL	Upper 95% CL	b	se(b)	OR	Lower 95% CL	Upper 95% CL
Family SES (Age Block 1):										
Low	.675	.574	1.964	.638	6.045	.283	.505	1.327	.493	3.573
Typical	.631	.520	1.879	.679	5.203	-.077	.437	1.080	.459	2.542
Family SES (Age Block 2):										
Low	--	--	--	--	--	.883	.508	2.417	.893	6.546
Typical	--	--	--	--	--	.409	.443	1.505	.631	3.589
Family SES (Age Block 3):										
Low	--	--	--	--	--	--	--	--	--	--
Typical	--	--	--	--	--	--	--	--	--	--
Race (Black)	-.075	.400	.928	.424	2.030	-.415	.319	.660	.353	1.234
Constant	-8.949					-6.542				
-2 Log Likelihood	249.784					347.175				

Continued on next page

Appendix 1 continued

% Correct Classification (Controls)	92.0					86.1
% Correct Classification (Full Model)	92.0					86.5
Model χ^2	21.44*					76.723*
Pseudo R^2 Controls only	.033					.224
Pseudo R^2 Full model	.102					.253
N	485					474

(Continues on next page)

Appendix I continued

Independent Variables:	MODEL 9: AGE BLOCK 4 on 1				
	b	*se(b)*	*OR*	Lower 95% CL	Upper 95% CL
Oppositional Defiant Problems	-.114	.082	.893	.760	1.049
Attention Deficit/Hyperactivity Problems	.015	.080	1.015	.868	1.187
Anxiety Problems	-.015	.065	.985	.867	1.120
Affective Problems	.054	.071	1.055	.919	1.212
Control Variables:					
Serious Theft (Age Block 2)	.013	.643	1.013	.287	3.576
	2.849	.538	17.266	6.012	49.584
Serious Theft (Age Block 3)	.255	.528	1.291	.458	3.634
	-.260	.708	.771	.193	3.086
Physical Aggression	.539*	.569	1.714	.572	5.138
Serious Violence (Age Block 2)					
Serious Violence (Age Block 3)					
Family SES (Age Block 1): Low	-.638	.871	.528	.096	2.910
	.732	.654	2.080	.577	7.494
	1.094	.827	2.985	.590	15.091
Typical	.160	.665	1.174	.319	4.319
Family SES (Age Block 2): Low	-.626	.777	.535	.117	2.393
	-.315	.606	.730	.223	2.454
Typical					
Family SES (Age Block 3): Low					
Typical					
Race (Black)	-.956	.485	.384	.149	.9594
Constant	-.253				
-2 Log Likelihood	163.512				
				Continued on next page	

Appendix I continued

% Correct Classification (Controls)	93.4				
% Correct Classification (Full Model)	92.5				
Model χ^2	55.529				
Pseudo R^2 Controls only	.279				
Pseudo R^2 Full model	.302				
N	440				

Note. CL = Confidence limit, 95% CL calculated as $\beta \pm (1.96$ standard error). SES = socioeconomic status.
$*p < .05.$

Appendix J: Logistic Regression Models 10-11: Effects of Teacher Reports of DSM-Oriented Problems at Age Block 2 on Serious Theft Behaviors at Age Blocks 3 and 4

	MODEL 10: AGE BLOCK 2 on 3					MODEL 11: AGE BLOCK 2 on 4				
Independent Variables:	b	se(b)	OR	Lower 95% CL	Upper 95% CL	b	se(b)	OR	Lower 95% CL	Upper 95% CL
Oppositional Defiant Problems	.065	.042	1.067	.982	1.160	.025	.066	1.026	.900	1.168
Attention Deficit/Hyperactivity Problems	.059	.039	1.061	.983	1.144	-.073	.070	.930	.811	1.065
Anxiety Problems	-.064	.038	.938	.871	1.010	.032	.057	1.032	.924	1.153
Affective Problems	.042	.039	1.043	.966	1.127	.063	.060	1.065	.947	1.198
Control Variables:										
Serious Theft (Age Block 2)	2.391*	.413	10.927	4.867	24.529	-.202	.650	.817	.228	2.923
Serious Theft (Age Block 3)	--	--	--	--	--	2.693*	.513	14.780	5.411	40.369
Physical Aggression Serious Violence (Age Block 2)										
Serious Violence (Age Block 3)										

Continued on next page

Appendix J continued

Independent Variables:	b	se(b)	OR	Lower 95% CL	Upper 95% CL	b	se(b)	OR	Lower 95% CL	Upper 95% CL
Family SES (Age Block 1):										
Low	.201	.516	1.222	.444	3.363	-.738	.856	.478	.089	2.559
Typical	-.072	.448	.931	.387	2.238	.409	.670	1.506	.405	5.596
Family SES (Age Block 2):										
Low	.948	.536	2.582	.903	7.381	1.272	.856	3.567	.667	19.076
Typical	.496	.469	1.642	.655	4.114	.460	.714	1.584	.391	6.415
Family SES (Age Block 3):										
Low	--	--	--	--	--	-.419	.785	.657	.141	3.063
Typical	--	--	--	--	--	-.194	.631	.824	.239	2.835
Race (Black)	-.526	.317	.591	.317	1.101	-1.174*	.479	.309	.121	.789
Constant	-8.519					-6.006				
-2 Log Likelihood	332.027					162.494				

Continued on next page

Appendix J continued

% Correct Classification (Controls)	85.3		93.6
% Correct Classification (Full Model)	86.1		93.6
Model χ^2	86.82*		50.73*
Pseudo R^2 Controls only	.192		.272
Pseudo R^2 Full model	.286		.284
N	469		436

Note. CL = Confidence limit, 95% CL calculated as $\beta \pm (1.96 \text{ standard error})$. SES = socioeconomic status.

*$p < .05$.

Appendix K: Logistic Regression Model 12: Effects of Teacher Reports of DSM-Oriented Problems at Age Block 3 on Serious Theft Behaviors at Age Block 4

Independent Variables:				Lower 95% CL	Upper 95% CL
	b	*se(b)*	*OR*		
Oppositional Defiant Problems	-.006	.067	.994	.872	1.134
Attention Deficit/Hyperactivity Problems	.062	.060	1.064	.946	1.197
Anxiety Problems	-.013	.049	.988	.897	1.087
Affective Problems	-.079	.057	.924	.826	1.034
Control Variables:					
Serious Theft (Age Block 2)	-.180	.651	.835	.233	2.992
Serious Theft (Age Block 3)	2.597*	.526	13.427	4.793	37.612
Physical Aggression Serious Violence (Age Block 2)					
Serious Violence (Age Block 3)					
Family SES (Age Block 1): Low	-.864	.866	.422	.077	2.301
	.291	.672	1.337	.358	4.995
	1.668*	.843	5.304	1.016	27.692
Typical	.633	.699	1.883	.478	7.414
Family SES (Age Block 2): Low	-.878	.813	.416	.084	2.046
	-.331	.656	.718	.199	2.596
Typical					
Family SES (Age Block 3): Low					
Typical					
Race (Black)	-1.238*	.478	.290	.114	.739

Continued on next page

Appendix K continued

Constant	-1.702				
-2 Log Likelihood	154.224				
% Correct Classification (Controls)	93.7				
% Correct Classification (Full Model)	93.9				
Model χ^2	52.48*				
Pseudo R^2 Controls only	.281				
Pseudo R^2 Full model	.301				
N	427				

Note. CL = Confidence limit, 95% CL calculated as $\beta \pm (1.96$ standard error). SES = socioeconomic status.
*$p < .05$.

Appendix L: Logistic Regression Models 13-15: Effect of Parent Reports of DSM-Oriented Problems at Age Block 1 on Serious Violent Behaviors at Age Blocks 2, 3, and 4

	MODEL 13: AGE BLOCK 2 on 1					MODEL 14: AGE BLOCK 3 on 1				
Independent Variables:	b	se(b)	OR	Lower 95% CL	Upper 95% CL	b	se(b)	OR	Lower 95% CL	Upper 95% CL
Oppositional Defiant Problems	.008	.040	1.008	.931	1.091	.053	.034	1.055	.986	1.128
Attention Deficit/Hyperactivity Problems	.013	.043	1.013	.930	1.103	-.020	.038	.980	.910	1.056
Anxiety Problems	.018	.048	1.018	.926	1.118	-.044	.044	.957	.877	1.044
Affective Problems	.054	.047	1.055	.963	1.156	.063	.040	1.065	.986	1.151
Control Variables:										
Physical Aggression (Age Block 1)	1.054*	.323	2.868	1.522	5.408	-.117	.298	.889	.496	1.594
Serious Violence (Age Block 2)	--	--	--	--	--	1.503*	.357	4.497	2.233	9.058
Serious Violence (Age Block 3)	--	--	--	--	--	--	--	--	--	--
Serious Theft (Age Block 2)	--	--	--	--	--	1.693*	.398	5.437	2.490	11.872
Serious Theft (Age Block 3)	--	--	--	--	--	--	--	--	--	--

Continued on next page

Appendix L continued

Independent Variables:	b	se(b)	OR	Lower 95% CL	Upper 95% CL	b	se(b)	OR	Lower 95% CL	Upper 95% CL
Family SES (Age Block 1):	.163	.479	1.178	.461	3.009	.320	.476	1.377	.542	3.496
Low	.131	.401	1.141	.519	2.504	.379	.397	1.461	.671	3.182
Typical										
Family SES (Age Block 2):	--	--	--	--	--	.955	.496	2.598	.984	6.861
Low	--	--	--	--	--	.795	.427	2.215	.960	5.114
Typical										
Family SES (Age Block 3):										
Low	--	--	--	--	--	--	--	--	--	--
Typical										
Race (Black)	1.189*	.389	3.285	1.532	7.043	.793*	.287	2.209	1.259	3.876
Constant	-8.518					-6.215				
-2 Log Likelihood	287.290					401.777				

Continued on next page

Appendix L continued

% Correct Classification (Controls)	89.9		82.7	
% Correct Classification (Full Model)	90.1		83.8	
Model χ^2		30.23*		81.805*
Pseudo R^2 Controls only		.103		.228
Pseudo R^2 Full model		.126		.248
N		485		475

(Continues on next page)

Appendix L continued

Independent Variables:	MODEL 15: AGE BLOCK 4 on 1				
	b	*se(b)*	*OR*	Lower 95% CL	Upper 95% CL
Oppositional Defiant Problems	.022	.053	1.022	.921	1.134
Attention Deficit/Hyperactivity Problems	.063	.058	1.065	.951	1.192
Anxiety Problems	-.145	.083	.863	.735	1.019
Affective Problems	.068	.061	1.0571	.950	1.207
Control Variables:					
Physical Aggression (Age Block 1)	-.252	.465	.777	.313	1.933
Serious Violence (Age Block 2)	-.401	.576	.670	.216	2.072
Serious Violence (Age Block 3)	1.530*	.447	4.619	1.922	11.100
Serious Theft (Age Block 2)	.138	.562	1.148	.381	3.457
Serious Theft (Age Block 3)	1.457*	.452	4.293	1.770	10.414
Family SES (Age Block 1): Low	.187	.866	1.206	.22	6.589
	1.517*	.688	4.559	1.184	17.559
Typical	.070	.748	1.073	.248	4.646
Family SES (Age Block 2): Low	-.799	.613	.450	.135	1.497
	-.776	.672	.460	.123	1.720
Typical	-.585	.551	.557	.189	1.643
Family SES (Age Block 3): Low					
Typical					
Race (Black)	.813	.453	2.254	.928	5.474

Continued on next page

Appendix L continued

Constant	-4.707				
-2 Log Likelihood	188.435				
% Correct Classification (Controls)	91.6				
% Correct Classification (Full Model)	91.6				
Model χ^2	50.14*				
Pseudo R^2 Controls only	.275				
Pseudo R^2 Full model	.299				
N	441				

Note. CL = Confidence limit, 95% CL calculated as $\beta \pm (1.96 \text{ standard error})$. SES = socioeconomic status.
*$p < .05$.

Appendix M: Logistic Regression Models 16-17: Effects of Parent Reports of DSM-Oriented Problems at Age Block 2 on Serious Violent Behaviors at Age Blocks 3 and 4

Independent Variables:	MODEL 16: AGE BLOCK 3 on 2					MODEL 17: AGE BLOCK 4 on 2				
	b	se(b)	OR	Lower 95% CL	Upper 95% CL	b	se(b)	OR	Lower 95% CL	Upper 95% CL
Oppositional Defiant Problems	.044	.033	1.045	.981	1.114	.071	.047	1.073	.978	1.178
Attention Deficit/Hyperactivity Problems	-.014	.037	.986	.917	1.059	.028	.055	1.028	.923	1.145
Anxiety Problems	-.032	.042	.969	.892	1.053	-.080	.063	.923	.804	1.060
Affective Problems	.076	.044	1.079	.990	1.176	.058	.063	1.059	.937	1.198
Control Variables:										
Physical Aggression (Age Block 1)	-.052	.297	.949	.530	1.699	-.234	.478	.792	.310	2.022
Serious Violence (Age Block 2)	1.492*	.357	4.447	2.208	8.957	-.465	.572	.628	.205	1.927
Serious Violence (Age Block 3)	--	--	--	--	--	1.365*	.462	3.917	1.583	9.692
Serious Theft (Age Block 2)	1.678	.399	5.357	2.453	11.703	.316	.557	1.371	.460	4.086
Serious Theft (Age Block 3)	--	--	--	--	--	1.475*	.465	4.371	1.756	10.876

Continued on next page

Appendix M continued

Independent Variables:	b	se(b)	OR	Lower 95% CL	Upper 95% CL	b	se(b)	OR	Lower 95% CL	Upper 95% CL
Family SES (Age Block 1):										
Low	.363	.480	1.438	.561	3.681	.414	.916	1.512	.251	9.108
Typical	.501	.405	1.650	.746	3.651	1.884*	.750	6.581	1.514	28.609
Family SES (Age Block 2):										
Low	1.039*	.494	2.827	1.074	7.445	.030	.720	1.031	.251	4.225
Typical	.769	.426	2.157	.936	4.968	-.956	.607	.384	.117	1.264
Family SES (Age Block 3):										
Low	--	--	--	--	--	-.732	.658	.481	.133	1.745
Typical	--	--	--	--	--	-.741	.546	.477	.164	1.389
Race (Black)	.822*	.287	2.274	1.296	3.990	1.112*	.480	3.041	1.188	7.784
Constant	-7.461					-8.773				
-2 Log Likelihood	411.704					179.210				

Continued on next page

Appendix M continued

% Correct Classification (Controls)	82.9		91.6
% Correct Classification (Full Model)	82.2		92.0
Model χ^2	85.965*		64.963*
Pseudo R^2 Controls only	.234		.280
Pseudo R^2 Full model	.261		.322
N	473		439

Note. CL = Confidence limit, 95% CL calculated as $\beta \pm (1.96$ standard error). SES = socioeconomic status.
*$p < .05$.

Appendix N: Logistic Regression Model 18: Effects of Parent Reports of DSM-Oriented Problems at Age Block 3 on Serious Violent Behaviors at Age Block 4

Independent Variables:	*MODEL 18: AGE BLOCK 3 on 4*				
				Lower 95%	Upper 95%
	b	*se(b)*	*OR*	CL	CL
Oppositional Defiant Problems	.075	.050	1.078	.977	1.190
Attention Deficit/Hyperactivity Problems	-.023	.060	.977	.869	1.100
Anxiety Problems	.040	.058	1.041	.929	1.166
Affective Problems	-.010	.060	.990	.880	1.113
Control Variables:					
Physical Aggression (Age Block 1)	-.410	.471	.664	.264	1.670
Serious Violence (Age Block 2)	-.025	.543	.975	.336	2.829
Serious Violence (Age Block 3)	1.937*	.418	6.941	3.057	15.762
Serious Theft (Age Block 2)					
Serious Theft (Age Block 3)					
Family SES (Age Block 1): Low	.239	.873	1.271	.230	7.033
	1.401*	.683	4.060	1.064	15.486
	.066	.743	1.068	.249	4.582
Typical	-.811	.606	.444	.135	1.457
Family SES (Age Block 2): Low	-.623	.649	.536	.150	1.912
	-.539	.524	.583	.209	1.628
Typical					
Family SES (Age Block 3): Low					
Typical					
				Continued on next page	

Appendix N continued

Independent Variables:	b	se(b)	OR	Lower 95% CL	Upper 95% CL
Race (Black)	.709	.447	2.032	.846	4.880
Constant	-8.194				
-2 Log Likelihood	199.936				
% Correct Classification (Controls) % Correct Classification (Full Model)	91.3 91.8				
Model χ^2	49.10*				
Pseudo R^2 Controls only Pseudo R^2 Full model	.220 .244				
N	439				

Note. CL = Confidence limit, 95% CL calculated as $\beta \pm (1.96 \text{ standard error})$. SES = socioeconomic status.
*$p < .05$.

Appendix O: Logistic Regression Models 19-21: Effects of Teacher Reports of DSM-Oriented Problems at Age Block 1 on Serious Violent Behaviors at Age Blocks 2, 3, and 4

	MODEL 19: AGE BLOCK 2 on 1					MODEL 20: AGE BLOCK 3 on 1				
Independent Variables:	b	se(b)	OR	Lower 95% CL	Upper 95% CL	b	se(b)	OR	Lower 95% CL	Upper 95% CL
Oppositional Defiant Problems	.075	.042	1.078	.992	1.172	.068	.036	1.071	.997	1.150
Attention Deficit/Hyperactivity Problems	-.015	.045	.985	.901	1.076	.039	.038	1.040	.966	1.120
Anxiety Problems	-.048	.043	.953	.876	1.038	-.060	.036	.942	.877	1.011
Affective Problems	.115*	.046	1.122	1.026	1.227	.085*	.038	1.089	1.010	1.174
Control Variables:										
Physical Aggression (Age Block 1)	.978*	.328	2.658	1.398	5.054	-.192	.303	.825	.455	1.495
Serious Violence (Age Block 2)	--	--	--	--	--	1.332*	.363	3.788	1.859	7.718
Serious Violence (Age Block 3)	--	--	--	--	--	--	--	--	--	--
Serious Theft (Age Block 2)	--	--	--	--	--	1.435	.401	4.201	1.915	9.216
Serious Theft (Age Block 3)	--	--	--	--	--	--	--	--	--	--

Continued on next page

Appendix O continued

Independent Variables:	b	se(b)	OR	Lower 95% CL	Upper 95% CL	b	se(b)	OR	Lower 95% CL	Upper 95% CL
Family SES (Age Block 1):										
Low	-.138	.489	.871	.334	2.273	.182	.477	1.200	.471	3.058
Typical	-.031	.414	.969	.430	2.182	.307	.403	1.359	.616	2.997
Family SES (Age Block 2):										
Low	--	--	--	--	--	.768	.504	2.154	.803	5.781
Typical	--	--	--	--	--	.778	.432	2.177	.933	5.080
Family SES (Age Block 3):										
Low	--	--	--	--	--	--	--	--	--	--
Typical	--	--	--	--	--	--	--	--	--	--
Race (Black)	.682	.401	1.979	.901	4.345	.144	.303	1.154	.637	2.092
Constant	-10.383					-10.472				
-2 Log Likelihood	275.160					378.104				

Continued on next page

Appendix O continued

% Correct Classification (Controls)	89.9			82.7	
% Correct Classification (Full Model)	89.7			81.9	
Model χ^2	42.36*			105.479*	
Pseudo R^2 Controls only	.103			.228	
Pseudo R^2 Full model	.174			.312	
N	485			475	

(Continues on next page)

Appendix O continued

Independent Variables:	MODEL 21: AGE BLOCK 4 on 1				
	b	se(b)	OR	Lower 95% CL	Upper 95% CL
Oppositional Defiant Problems	.104	.057	1.110	.991	1.242
Attention Deficit/Hyperactivity Problems	-.052	.062	.949	.841	1.071
Anxiety Problems	-.087	.063	.917	.811	1.036
Affective Problems	-.019	.064	.981	.865	1.113
Control Variables:					
Physical Aggression (Age Block 1)	-.209	.467	.811	.325	2.027
Serious Violence (Age Block 2)	-.424	.588	.654	.207	2.072
Serious Violence (Age Block 3)	1.614*	.469	5.023	2.005	12.583
Serious Theft (Age Block 2)	-.052	.572	.949	.309	2.913
Serious Theft (Age Block 3)	1.480*	.457	4.393	1.794	10.757
Family SES (Age Block 1): Low	.222	.885	1.249	.220	7.081
	1.438*	.695	4.211	1.078	16.453
	-.151	.752	.860	.197	3.753
Typical	-.808	.617	.446	.133	1.493
Family SES (Age Block 2): Low	-.813	.661	.443	.121	1.618
	-.625	.561	.535	.178	1.606
Typical					
Family SES (Age Block 3): Low					
Typical					
Race (Black)	.586	.487	1.797	.691	4.668
Constant	-1.011				
					Continued on next page

Appendix O continued

-2 Log Likelihood	187.840				
% Correct Classification (Controls)	91.6				
% Correct Classification (Full Model)	91.8				
Model χ^2	61.535*				
Pseudo R^2 Controls only	.275				
Pseudo R^2 Full model	.302				
N	441				

Note. CL = Confidence limit, 95% CL calculated as $\beta \pm (1.96$ standard error). SES = socioeconomic status.
*$p < .05$.

Appendix P: Logistic Regression Models 22-23: Effects of Teacher Reports of DSM-Oriented Problems at Age Block 2 on Serious Violent Behaviors at Age Blocks 3 and 4

Independent Variables:	MODEL 22: AGE BLOCK 3 on 2					MODEL 23: AGE BLOCK 4 on 2				
	b	se(b)	OR	Lower 95% CL	Upper 95% CL	b	se(b)	OR	Lower 95% CL	Upper 95% CL
Oppositional Defiant Problems	.035	.038	1.035	.960	1.116	.102	.057	1.108	.990	1.239
Attention Deficit/Hyperactivity Problems	.071*	.036	1.074	1.001	1.152	-.042	.054	.959	.862	1.066
Anxiety Problems	-.011	.034	.989	.926	1.056	-.036	.055	.965	.866	1.076
Affective Problems	.039	.036	1.039	.969	1.115	.051	.059	1.052	.937	1.180
Control Variables:										
Physical Aggression (Age Block 1)	-.113	.298	.893	.497	1.602	-.165	.465	.848	.341	2.107
Serious Violence (Age Block 2)	1.288*	.377	3.627	1.733	7.590	-.623	.618	.536	.160	1.800
Serious Violence (Age Block 3)	--	--	--	--	--	1.416*	.471	4.122	1.636	10.385
Serious Theft (Age Block 2)	1.547	.409	4.699	2.107	10.477	.355	.557	1.427	.479	4.249
Serious Theft (Age Block 3)	--	--	--	--	--	1.432*	.483	4.185	1.624	10.787

Continued on next page

Appendix P continued

Independent Variables:	b	se(b)	OR	Lower 95% CL	Upper 95% CL	b	se(b)	OR	Lower 95% CL	Upper 95% CL
Family SES (Age Block 1):										
Low	.157	.484	1.170	.453	3.021	.173	.891	1.189	.207	6.820
Typical	.261	.403	1.298	.589	2.859	1.599*	.700	4.946	1.255	19.487
Family SES (Age Block 2):										
Low	.753	.518	2.123	.770	5.854	-.262	.748	.769	.178	3.331
Typical	.844	.442	2.325	.977	5.531	-1.034	.612	.356	.107	1.180
Family SES (Age Block 3):										
Low	--	--	--	--	--	-1.082	.668	.339	.091	1.255
Typical	--	--	--	--	--	-.754	.543	.471	.162	1.365
Race (Black)	.295	.299	1.343	.747	2.415	.484	.481	1.622	.632	4.165
Constant	-10.691					-8.014				
-2 Log Likelihood	370.268					179.789				

Appendix P continued

% Correct Classification (Controls)	82.8	92.2
% Correct Classification (Full Model)	82.8	92.0
Model χ^2	105.602*	64.051*
Pseudo R^2 Controls only	.223	.292
Pseudo R^2 Full model	.316	.319
N	470	437

Note. CL = Confidence limit, 95% CL calculated as $\beta \pm (1.96$ standard error). SES = socioeconomic status.
*$p < .05$.

Appendix Q: Logistic Regression Model 24: Effects of Teacher Reports of DSM-Oriented Problems at Age Block 3 on Serious Violent Behaviors at Age Block 4

Independent Variables:	*MODEL 24: AGE BLOCK 3 on 4*				
	b	*se(b)*	*OR*	Lower 95% CL	Upper 95% CL
Oppositional Defiant Problems	.158*	.057	1.171	1.047	1.309
Attention Deficit/Hyperactivity Problems	-.026	.050	.975	.883	1.076
Anxiety Problems	-.052	.039	.949	.879	1.025
Affective Problems	-.011	.046	.989	.905	1.082
Control Variables:					
Physical Aggression (Age Block 1)	-.247	.453	.781	.321	1.897
Serious Violence (Age Block 2)	.207	.554	1.229	.415	3.643
Serious Violence (Age Block 3)	1.643*	.448	5.169	2.150	12.432
Serious Theft (Age Block 2)					
Serious Theft (Age Block 3)					
Family SES (Age Block 1): Low	.388	.877	1.474	.264	8.228
	1.529*	.704	4.615	1.162	18.333
	-.404	.772	.668	.147	3.032
Typical	-1.035	.633	.355	.103	1.228
Family SES (Age Block 2): Low	-1.124	.697	.325	.083	1.275
	-.923	.572	.397	.129	1.220
Typical					
Family SES (Age Block 3): Low					
Typical					
Race (Black)	.227	.451	1.255	.518	3.040
Continued on next page					

Appendix Q continued

Constant	-7.371				
-2 Log Likelihood	186.149				
% Correct Classification (Controls)	91.8				
% Correct Classification (Full Model)	91.6				
Model χ^2	56.17*				
Pseudo R^2 Controls only	.218				
Pseudo R^2 Full model	.285				
N	428				

Note. CL = Confidence limit, 95% CL calculated as $\beta \pm (1.96$ standard error). SES = socioeconomic status.
*$p < .05$.

References

Abikoff, H., & Klein, R. G. (1992). Attention-deficit hyperactivity and conduct disorder: Co-morbidity and implications for treatment. *Journal of Consulting and Clinical Psychology, 60,* 881-892.

Achenbach, T. M. (1985). *Assessment and taxonomy of child and adolescent psychopathology.* Newbury Park, CA: Sage Publications.

Achenbach, T. M. (1997). *Manual for the Young Adult Self-Report and Young Adult Behavior Checklist.* Burlington, VT: University of Vermont, Department of Psychiatry.

Achenbach, T. M. (2001). Challenges and benefits of assessment, diagnostic, and taxonomy for clinical practice and research. *Australian and New Zealand Journal of Psychiatry, 35,* 263-271.

Achenbach, T. M. (2005a). Advancing assessment of children and adolescents: Commentary on evidence-based assessment of child and adolescent disorders. *Journal of Clinical Child and Adolescent Psychology, 34,* 541-547.

Achenbach, T. M. (2005b). *Later developments.* Burlington, VT: University of Vermont, Research Center for Children, Youth, & Families. Retrieved August 11, 2005, from http://www.aseba.org/ABOUTUS/later_developments.html

Achenbach, T. M. (2006). As others see us – Clinical and research implications of cross-informant correlations for psychopathology. *Current Directions in Psychological Science, 15*(2), 94-98.

Achenbach, T. M., Bernstein, A., & Dumenci, L. (2005). A snark or a boojum? Exploring multitaxonomic possibilities and building on Widiger's commentary. *Journal of Personality Assessment, 84*(4), 66-69.

Achenbach, T. M., & Dumenci, L. (2001). Advances in empirically-based assessment: Revised cross-informant syndromes and new DSM-oriented scales for the CBCL, YSR, and TRF: Comment on Lengua, Sadowski, Friedrich, & Fisher. *Journal of Consulting and Clinical Psychology, 69*(4), 699-702.

Achenbach, T. M., Dumenci, L., & Rescorla, L. A. (2000). *Ratings of the relations between DSM-IV diagnostic categories and items on the CBCL/1 ½ -5 and C-TRF.* Burlington, VT: University of Vermont, Research Center for Children, Youth, & Families. Retrieved August 11, 2005, from http://www.aseba.org/

Achenbach, T. M., Dumenci, L., & Rescorla, L. A. (2001). *Ratings of relations between DSM-IV diagnostic categories and items of the CBCL/6-18, TRF, and YSR.* Burlington, VT: University of Vermont, Research Center for Children, Youth, & Families. Retrieved August 11, 2005, from http://www.aseba.org/

Achenbach, T. M., Dumenci, L., & Rescorla, L. A. (2002). Ten-year comparisons of problems and competencies for national samples of youth: Self, parent, and teacher reports. *Journal of Emotional and Behavioral Disorders, 10*(4), 194-213.

Achenbach, T. M., & Edelbrock, C. S. (1983). *Manual for the Child Behavior Checklist and Revised Child Behavior Profile.* Burlington, VT: University of Vermont, Department of Psychiatry.

Achenbach, T. M., & Edelbrock, C. S. (1987). *Manual for the Youth Self-Report and Profile.* Burlington, VT: University of Vermont, Department of Psychiatry.

Achenbach, T. M., McConaughy, S. H., & Howell, C. T. (1987). Child/adolescent behavioral and emotional problems: Implications of cross-informant correlations for situational specificity. *Psychological Bulletin, 101*, 213-232.

Achenbach, T. M., & Rescorla, L. A. (2001). Manual for the ASEBA School-Age Forms and Profiles: An Integrated System for Multi-Informant Assessment. Burlington, VT: University of Vermont.

Agresti, A., & Finlay, B. (1997). *Statistical methods for the social sciences.* Upper Saddle River, NJ: Prentice Hall.

Allison, P. D. (1999). Comparing logit and probit coefficients across groups. *Sociological Methods & Research, 28*(2), 186-208.

American Academy of Child and Adolescent Psychiatry (1998). Work Group on Quality Issues: Practice parameters for the assessment and treatment of children and adolescents with depressive disorders. *Journal of the American Academy of Child and Adolescent Psychiatry, 37*(Suppl. 10), 63S-83S.

American Psychiatric Association (2000). *Diagnostic and statistical manual of mental disorders* (4th ed., text rev.). Washington, DC: Author.

Anderson, J. C., & McGee, R. (1994). Comorbidity of depression in children and adolescents. In W. M. Reynolds & H. F. Johnson (Eds.), *Handbook of depression in children and adolescents* (pp. 581-601). New York: Plenum.

Anderson, J.C., Williams, S., McGee, R., & Silva, P.A. (1987). DSM-III disorders in preadolescent children: Prevalence in a large sample from the general population. *Archives of General Psychiatry, 44*, 69-76.

Andrews, D.A., & Bonta, J. (2003). *The psychology of criminal conduct (3rd edition).* Cincinnati, OH: Anderson Publishing.

Angermeyer, M. C., Cooper, B., & Link, B. G. (1998). Mental disorder and violence: Results of epidemiological studies in the era of de-institutionalization. *Social Psychiatry and Psychiatric Epidemiology, 33*, S1-S6.

Angold, A., & Costello, E. J. (1993). Depressive comorbidity in children and adolescents: Empirical, theoretical, and methodological issues. *American Journal of Psychiatry, 150*, 1779-1791.

Angold, A., Costello, E. J., & Erkanli, A. (1999). Comorbidity. *Journal of Child Psychology and Psychiatry and Allied Disciplines, 40*, 57-87.

Anxiety Disorders Association of America (2006). *Brief Overview of Anxiety Disorders.* Retrieved March 1, 2006, from http:www.adaa.org/GettingHelp/BriefOverview.asp.

August, G.J., Realmuto, G.M., Joyce, T., & Hektner, J.M. (1999). Persistence and desistence of oppositional defiant disorder in a community sample of children with ADHD. *Journal of the American Academy of Child and Adolescent Psychiatry, 38*, 1262-1270.

Bachman, R., & Paternoster, R. (2004). *Statistics for criminology and criminal justice.* Boston: McGraw Hill.

Ballenger, J. C., Davidson, J. R., Lecrubier, Y., Nutt, D. J., Bobes, J., Beidel, D. C., Ono, Y., & Westenberg, H. G. (1998). Consensus statement on social anxiety disorder from the International Consensus Group on Depression and Anxiety. *Journal of Clinical Psychiatry, 59*(Suppl. 17), 54-60.

Barkley, R.A. (1996). Attention-deficit hyperactivity disorder. In E.J. Mash and R.A. Barkley (Eds.), *Child psychopathology* (pp. 63-112). New York: Guilford Press.

Barkley, R.A. (1998). *Attention-deficit hyperactivity disorder: A handbook of diagnosis and treatment* (2nd ed.). New York: Guilford Press.

Barlow, D., & Durand, V. (2002). Abnormal psychology: An integrative approach (3rd ed.). Belmont, CA: Wadsworth/Thomson Learning.

Bartol, C. R., & Bartol, A. M. (2005). *Criminal behavior: A psychosocial approach.* Upper Saddle River, NJ: Pearson Prentice Hall.

Barak, G. (2003). *Violence and nonviolence: Pathways to understanding.* Thousand Oaks, CA: Sage Publications.

Bauer, L. O., & Houston, R. J. (2004). Neurophysiological and cognitive correlates of antisocial behavior. In D. H. Fishbein (Ed.), *The science, treatment, and prevention of antisocial behaviors* (Vol. II, pp. 5/1-28). Kingston, NJ: Civic Research Institute.

Beitchman, J. H., Wekerle, C., & Hood, J. (1987). Diagnostic continuity from preschool to middle childhood. *Journal of the American Academy of Child and Adolescent Psychiatry, 26*, 694-699.

Benson, M.L. (2002). *Crime and the life course: An introduction.* Los Angeles: Roxbury Publishing Company.

Beyers, J. M., & Loeber, R. (2003). Untangling developmental relations between depressed mood and delinquency in male adolescents. *Journal of Abnormal Child Psychology, 31*(3), 247-266.

Biederman, J., Mick, E., Faraone, S. V., & Burback, M. (2001). Patterns of remission and symptom decline in conduct disorder: A four-year prospective study of an ADHD sample. *Journal of the American Academy of Child and Adolescent Psychiatry, 40*, 290-298.

Birmaher, B., Ryan, N. D., Williamson, D. E., Brent, D. A., Kaufman, J., Daul, R. E., Perel, J., & Nelson, B. (1996). Childhood and adolescent depression: A review of the past 10 years. Part I. *Journal of the American Academy of Child and Adolescent Psychiatry, 29*, 914-918.

Blaauw, E., Arensman, E., Kraaij, V., Winkel, F. W., & Bout, R. (2002). *Mentally disordered offenders: International perspectives on assessment and treatment.* The Hague: Elsevier.

Blum, R. W., Beuhring, T., Shew, M. L., Bearinger, L. H., Sieving, R. W., & Resnick, M. D. (2000). The effects of race/ethnicity, income, and family structure on adolescent risk behaviors. *American Journal of Public Health, 90*, 1879-1884.

Blumberg, S. H., & Izard, C. E. (1985). Affective and cognitive characteristics of depression in 10- and 11- year-old children. *Journal of Personality and Social Psychology, 49*, 194-202.

Blumstein, A., Cohen, J., Roth, J. A., & Visher, C. A. (Eds.). *Criminal careers and "career criminals."* Washington, DC: National Academy of Sciences.

Blumstein, A., Farrington, D. P., & Moitra, S. D. (1985). Delinquency careers: Innocents, desisters, and persisters. In M. Tonry & N. Morris (Eds.), *Crime and justice: An annual review of research* (Vol. 6, pp. 137-168). Chicago: University of Chicago Press.

Boesky, L. M. (2002). *Juvenile offenders with mental health disorders: Who are they and what do we do with them?* Lanham, MD: American Correctional Association.

Bond, L. A., & Compas, B. E. (Eds.). (1989). *Primary prevention and promotion in the schools.* Newbury Park, CA: Sage Publications.

Bonta, J., Law, M., & Hanson, R. K. (1998). The prediction of criminal and violent recidivism among mentally disordered offenders: A meta-analysis. *Psychological Bulletin, 123*, 123-142.

Brame, R., Paternoster, R., Mazerolle, P., & Piquero, A. (1998). Testing for the equality of maximum-likelihood regression coefficients between two independent equations. *Journal of Quantitative Criminology, 14*(3), 245-261.

Brady, E. U., & Kendall, P. C. (1992). Comorbidity of anxiety and depression in children and adolescents. *Psychological Bulletin, 111*, 244-255.

Brawman-Mintzer, O., & Lydiard, R. B. (1996). Generalized anxiety disorder: Issues in epidemiology. *Journal of Clinical Psychiatry, 57*(Suppl. 7), 3-8.

Broidy, L. M., Nagin, D. S., Tremblay, R. E., Bates, J. E., Brame, B., Dodge, K. A., Fergusson, D., Horwood, J. L., Loeber, R., Laird, R., Lynam, D. R., Moffitt, T. E., Pettit, G. S., & Vitaro, F. (2003). Developmental trajectories of childhood disruptive behaviors and adolescent delinquency: A six-site, cross-national study. *Developmental Psychology, 39*, 222-245.

Brown, R.M. (1979). Historical patterns of violence. In H. D. Graham & T. R. Gurr (Eds.), *Violence in America: Historical and comparative perspectives* (Vol. 1, pp. 35-64). Washington, DC: U.S. Government Printing Office.

Brownhill, S., Wilhelm, K., Barclay, L., & Schmied, V. (2005). 'Build big': Hidden depression in men. *Australian and New Zealand Journal of Psychiatry, 39*, 921-931.

Bry, B. H. (1982). Reducing the incidence of adolescent problems through preventive intervention: One- and five-year follow-up. *American Journal of Community Psychology, 10*, 265-276.

Burke, J. D., Loeber, R., Mutchka, J. S., & Lahey, B. B. (2002). A question for DSM-V: Which better predicts persistent conduct disorder – Delinquent acts or conduct symptoms? *Criminal Behavior and Mental Health, 12*, 37-52.

Burns, M. K., Costello, E. J., Angold, A., Tweed, D., Stangl, D., Farmer, E. M., & Erkanli, A. (1995). Children's mental health service use across service sectors. *Health Affairs, 14*, 147-159.

Butterfield, F. (1996). *All god's children: The Bosket family and the American tradition of violence.* New York: Avon Books.

Campbell, S. B. (1995). Behavioral problems in preschool children: A review of recent research. *Journal of Child Psychology and Psychiatry and Allied Disciplines, 36,* 113-149.

Campbell, S. B., & Ewing, L. J. (1990). Hard-to-manage preschoolers: Adjustment at age nine and predictors of continuing symptoms. *Journal of Child Psychology and Psychiatry, 31,* 871-889.

Carlson, C. I., Tharinger, D. J., Bricklin, P. M., DeMers, S. T., & Paavola, J. C. (1996). Health care reform and psychological practice in schools. *Professional Psychology: Research and Practice, 27*(1), 14-23.

Caspi, A. (2000). The child is father of the man: Personality continuities from childhood to adulthood. *Journal of Personality and Social Psychology, 78,* 158-172.

Caspi, A., & Moffitt, T. E. (1995). The continuity of maladaptive behavior: From description to understanding in the study of antisocial behavior. In D. Cicchetti & D. J. Cohen (Eds.), *Developmental Psychopathology* (Vol. 2, pp. 472-511). New York: Wiley Press.

Catalano, R. F., Arthur, M. W., Hawkins, J. D., Berglund, L., & Olson, J. J. (1998). Comprehensive community- and school-based interventions to prevent antisocial behavior. In R. Loeber & D. P. Farrington (Eds.), *Serious & violent juvenile offenders* (pp.248-283). Thousand Oaks, CA: Sage Publications.

Cauce, A. M., Comer, J. P., & Schwartz, D. (1987). Long-term effects of a systems-oriented school prevention program. *American Journal of Orthopsychiatry, 57,* 127-131.

Clarke, R. V. (1995). Situational crime prevention. In M. Tonry & D. P. Farrington (Eds.), *Crime and justice: A review of research* (Vol. 19, pp. 91-150). Chicago: University of Chicago Press.

Clogg, C. C., Petkova, E., & Haritou, A. (1995). Symposium on applied regression: Statistical methods for comparing regression coefficients between models. *American Journal of Sociology, 100*(5), 1261-1293.

Cochran, S. V., & Rabinowitz, F. E. (2000). *Men and depression.* San Diego, CA: Academic Press.

Cocozza, J. J., Melick, M. E., & Steadman, H. J. (1978). Trends in violent crime among ex-mental patients. *Criminology, 161,* 317-334.

Cocozza, J. J., & Skowyra, K. (2000). Youth with mental health disorders: Issues and emerging responses. *Juvenile Justice, 7*(1), 4-13.

Cocozza, J. J., Veysey, B. M., Chapin, D. A., Dembo, R., Walters, W., & Farina, S. (2005). Diversion from the juvenile justice system: The Miami-Dade Juvenile Assessment Center Post-Arrest Diversion Program. *Substance Use & Misuse, 40*, 935-951.

Cohen, J. (1986). Research on criminal careers: Individual frequency rates and offense seriousness. In A. Blumstein, J. Cohen, J. A. Roth, & C. A. Visher (Eds.), *Criminal careers and "career criminals"* (Vol. 1, pp. 292-418). Washington, DC: National Academy Press.

Cohen, J A.., Mannarino, A. P., Murray, L. K., & Igelman, R. (2006). Psychosocial interventions for maltreated and violence-exposed children. *Journal of Social Issues, 62*(4), 737-766.

Cohen, P., Cohen, J., & Brook, J. (1993), An epidemiological study of disorders in late childhood and adolescence-II. Persistent disorders. *Journal of Child Psychology and Psychiatry, 34*, 869-877.

Cohen, P., Cohen, J., Kasen, S., Velez, C. N., Hartmark, C., Johnson, J., Rojas, M., Brook, J., Streuning, E. L. (1993). An epidemiological study of disorders in late childhood and adolescence: I. Age and gender-specific prevalence. *Journal of Child Psychiatry and Psychology, 34*, 851-867.

Cohen, R., Parmelee, D. X., Irwin, L, Weisz, J. R., Howard, P., Purcell, P., & Best, A. M. (1990). Characteristics of children and adolescents in a psychiatric hospital and a corrections facility. *Journal of the American Academy of Child and Adolescent Psychiatry, 29*, 909-913.

Comer, J. P. (1988). Educating poor minority children. *Scientific American, 259*, 42-48.

Comer, R. J. (2004). *Abnormal psychology (*5th ed.*).* New York: Worth.

Conduct Problems Prevention Research Group (2002). Evaluation of the first 3 years of the Fast Track Prevention Trial with children at high risk for adolescent conduct problems. *Journal of Abnormal Child Psychology, 30*(1), 9-35.

Connor, D. F. (2002). Aggression and antisocial behavior in children and adolescents: Research and treatment. New York: Guilford Press.

Connor, D. F., Carlson, G. A., Chang, K.D., Daniolos, P. T., Ferziger, R., Findling, R. L., Hutchinson, J. G., Malone, R. P., Halperin, J. M., Plattner, B., Post, R. M., Reynolds, D. L., Rogers, K. M., Saxena, K., & Steiner, H. (2006). Juvenile maladaptive aggression: A review of prevention, treatment, and service configuration and a proposed research agenda. *Journal of Clinical Psychiatry, 67*(5), 808-820.

Connor, D. F., & Steingard, R. J. (1996). A clinical approach to the pharmacotherapy of aggression in children and adolescents. *Annals of the New York Academy of Sciences, 794*, 290-307.

Cook, P. J., & Laub, J. H. (2002). After the epidemic: Recent trend in youth violence in the United States. In M. Tonry & M. H. Moore (Eds.), *Youth violence* (pp. 27-64). Chicago: University of Chicago Press.

Costello, E. J., Angold, A., Burns, B. J., Stangl, D. K., Tweed, D. L., Erkanli, A., & Worthman, C. M. (1996). The Great Smoky Mountains Study of Youth: Goals, design, methods, and the prevalence of DSM-III-R disorders. *Archives of General Psychiatry, 53,* 1129-1136.

Cowley, G. (1993, July 26). The not-young and the restless. *Newsweek*, 48-49.

Cronbach, L. J. (1951). Coefficient alpha and the internal structure of tests. *Psychometrika, 16,* 297-334.

Curran, D. J., & Renzetti, C. M. (2001). *Theories of crime.* Boston: Allyn and Bacon.

Davis, D. L., Bean, Jr., G. J., Schumacher, J. E., & Stringer, T. L., (1991). Prevalence of emotional disorders in a juvenile justice institutional population. *American Journal of Forensic Psychology, 9*(1), 5-17.

Dembo, R., Cervenka, K. A., Hunter, B., Wang, W. (1999). Engaging high risk families in community based intervention services. *Aggression and Violent Behavior, 4*(1), 41-58.

Dembo, R., Dudell, G., Livingston, S., & Schmeidler, J. (2001). Family empowerment intervention: Conceptual foundations and clinical practices. *Family Empowerment as an Intervention Strategy in Juvenile Delinquency,* 1-31.

Dembo, R., Schmeidler, J., Seeberger, W., Shemwell, M., Rollie, M., Pacheco, K., Livingston, S., & Wothke, W. (2001). Long-term impact of a family empowerment intervention on a juvenile offender psychosocial functioning. *Family Empowerment as an Intervention Strategy in Juvenile Delinquency,* 59-109.

Dembo, R., Seeberger, W., Shemwell, M., Klein, L., Rollie, M., Pacheco, K., Schmeidler, J., Hartsfield, A., & Wothke, W. (2000). Psychosocial functioning among juvenile offender 12 months after family empowerment intervention. *Journal of Offender Rehabilitation, 32*(1/2), 1-56.

Dembo, R., Shemwell, M., Guida, J., Schmeidler, J., Pacheco, K., & Seeberger, W. (1998). A longitudinal study of the impact of a family empowerment intervention on juvenile offender psychosocial functioning: A first assessment. *Journal of Child & Adolescent Substance Abuse, 8*(1), 15-54.

Dembo, R., Turner, G., Borden, P., Schmeidler, J., & Manning, D. (1995). Screening high risk youths for potential problems: Field application in the use of the Problem Oriented Screening Instrument for Teenagers (POSIT). *Journal of Child & Adolescent Substance Abuse, 3,* 69-93.

Dembo, R., Williams, L., La Voie, L., Getreu, A., Berry, E., Genung, A., Schmeidler, J., Wish, E., & Kern, J. (1990). A longitudinal study of the relationships among alcohol use, marijuana/hashish use, cocaine use and emotional/psychological functioning problems in a cohort of high risk youths. *International Journal of the Addictions, 25,* 1341-1382.

Dembo, R., Williams, L., Wish, E. D., & Schmeidler, J. (1990). *Urine testing of detained juveniles to identify high-risk youth.* Washington, DC: U.S. Department of Justice.

Dembo, R., Wothke, W., Seeberger, W., Shemwell, M., Pacheco, K., Rollie, M., Schmeidler, J., Klein, L., Hartsfield, A., & Livingston, S. (2000). Testing a model of the influence of family problem factors on high-risk youths' troubled behavior: A three-wave longitudinal study. *Journal of Psychoactive Drugs, 32*(1), 55-65.

Duhig, A. M., & Phares, V. (2003). Adolescents', mothers', and fathers' perspectives of emotional and behavioral problems: Distress, Control, and Motivation to Change. *Child & Family Behavioral Therapy, 25*(4), 39-52.

Duhig, A. M., Renk, K., Epstein, M. K., & Phares, V. (2000). Interparental agreement on internalizing, externalizing, and total behavior problems: A meta-analysis. *Clinical Psychology: Science and Practice, 7*, 435-453.

Dunford, F, & Elliott, D. (1984). Identifying career offenders using self-reported data. *Journal of Research in Crime and Delinquency, 21*, 57-87.

Durlak, J. A. (1995). School-based prevention programs for children and adolescents. *Developmental clinical psychology and psychiatry.* Thousand Oaks, CA: Sage Publications.

Earls, F. (1980). The prevalence of behavior problems in 3-year-old children. *Archives of General Psychiatry, 37*, 1153-1159.

Edelbrock, C. S., & Achenbach, T. M. (1984). The teacher version of the Child Behavior Profile: 1. Boys aged six through eleven. *Journal of Consulting and Clinical Psychology, 52,* 207-217.

Elder, G. H. (1979). Historical change in life patterns and personality. In P. Baltes & O. Brim, Jr. (Eds.), *Life-span development and behavior* (pp. 117-159). New York: Academic Press.

Elder, G. H. (1985). Perspectives on the Life-Course. In G. H. Elder (Ed.), *Life course dynamics* (pp. 23-49). Ithaca, NY: Cornell University Press.

Elliott, D.S. (1994). Serious violent offenders: Onset, developmental course, and termination. *Criminology, 32*, 1-23.

Elliott, D.S. (2000). Violent offending over the life course: A sociological perspective. In N. A. Krasnegor, N. B. Anderson, & D. R. Bynum (Eds.), *Health and behavior* (Vol. 1, pp. 189-204). Rockville, MD: National Institutes of Health, Office of Behavioral and Social Sciences.

Elliott, D. S., & Ageton, S. S. (1980). Reconciling race and class differences in self-reported and official estimates of delinquency. *American Sociological Review, 45*(1), 95-110.

Elliott, D. S., Huizinga, D., & Ageton, S. S. (1985). *Explaining delinquency and drug use.* Beverly Hills, CA: Sage.

Elliott, D. S., Huizinga, D., & Morse, B. (1986). Self-reported violent offending: A descriptive analysis of juvenile violent offenders and their offending careers. *Journal of Interpersonal Violence, 1*, 472-514.

Elliott D. S., & Voss, H. L. (1974). *Delinquency and dropout.* Lexington, MA : D.C. Health.

Eron, L. D., Huesmann, L. R., Dubow, E., Romanoff, R., & Yarmel, P. W. (1987). Aggression and its correlates. In D. H. Crowell, I. M., Evans, & C. R. O'Donnell (Eds.), *Childhood aggression and violence* (pp. 249-262). New York: Plenum.

Esbensen, F. (2004). Youth violence: An overview. In M.A. Zahn, H.H. Brownstein, and S.L. Jackson (Eds.), *Violence: From theory to research* (pp. 177-193). Cincinnati, OH: Anderson Publishing/LexisNexis.

Fabio, A., Loeber, R., Balasubramani, G. K., Roth, J., Fu, W. J., & Farrington, D. P. (2006). Why some generations are more violent than others: Assessment of age, period, and cohort effects. *Journal of American Epidemiology, 164*(2), 151-160.

Farrington, D. P. (1986). Age and crime. In M. Tonry & N. Morris (Eds.), *Crime and Justice Review* (pp. 29-90). Chicago: University of Chicago Press.

Farrington, D. P. (1989). Early predictors of adolescent aggression and adult violence. *Violence and Victims, 4*, 79-100.

Farrington, D. P. (1995). The development of offending and antisocial behavior from childhood: Key findings from the Cambridge study in delinquency development. *Journal of Child Psychology & Psychiatry, 360*, 929-964.

Farrington, D. P. (2005). *Integrated developmental & life-course theories of offending: Advances in Criminological Theory* (Vol. 14). New Brunswick, NJ: Transaction Publishers.

Farrington, D. P., Loeber, R., Stouthamer-Loeber, M., Van Kammen, W. B., & Schmidt, L. (1996). Self-reported delinquency and a combined delinquency seriousness scale based on boys, mothers, and teachers: Concurrent and predictive validity for African-Americans and Caucasians. *Criminology, 34*, 493-517.

Farrington, D. P., Loeber, R., & Van Kammen, W. B. (1990). Long-term criminal outcomes of hyperactivity-impulsivity-attention deficit and conduct problems in childhood. In L. Robins & M. Rutter (Eds.), *Straight and devious pathways from childhood to adulthood* (pp. 62-81). New York: Cambridge University Press.

Farrington, D. P., & West, D. J. (1990). The Cambridge Study in Delinquent Development. In H. J. Kerner & G. Kaiser (Eds.), *Criminality: Personality, behavior and life history* (pp. 115-138). Berlin: Springer-Verlag.

Farrington, D. P., & West, D. J. (1993). Criminal, penal, and life histories of life offenders: Risk and protective factors and early identification. *Criminal Behaviour and Mental Health, 3*, 492-523.

Fergusson, D. M., & Horwood, L. J. (1995). Predictive validity of categorically and dimensionally scored measures of disruptive childhood behaviors. *Journal of the American Academy of Child and Adolescent Psychiatry, 34*, 477-485.

Fergusson, D. M., Horwood, L. J., & Lynskey, M. (1994). The childhoods of multiple problem adolescents: A 15-year longitudinal study. *Journal of Child Psychology and Psychiatry and Allied Discipline, 35*, 1123-1140.

Fergusson, D. M., Horwood, L. J., Ridder, E. M., & Beautrais, A. L. (2005). Subthreshold depression in adolescence and mental health outcomes in adulthood. *Archives of General Psychiatry, 62*, 66-72.

Fleming, J. E., & Offord, D. R. (1990). Epidemiology of childhood depressive disorders: A critical review. *Journal of the American Academy of Child and Adolescent Psychiatry, 29*, 571-580.

Flynn, L. M. (1987). The stigma of mental illness. In A.B. Hatfield (Ed.), *Families of the mentally ill: Meeting the challenges* (pp. 53-60). San Francisco: Jossey-Bass.

Foley, H. A., Carlton, C. O., & Howell, R. J. (1996). The relationship of attention deficit hyperactivity disorder and conduct disorder to juvenile delinquency: Legal implications. *Bulletin of the American Academy of Psychiatry and Law, 24*, 333-345.

Fong, G., Frost, D., & Stansfeld, S (2001). Road rage: A psychiatric phenomenon? *Social Psychiatry and Psychiatric Epidemiology, 36*, 277-286.

Fox, J. A. & Zawitz, M. W. (2000, March). *Homicide trends in the United States: 2002 update.* (Crime Data Brief NCJ 179767). U.S. Department of Justice, Office of Justice Programs.

Frances, A. J., Pincus, H. A., Widiger, T. A., Davis, W. W., & First, M. B. (1990). DSM-IV: Work in progress. *American Journal of Psychiatry, 147*, 1439-1448.

Frick, P. J. (1998). Conduct disorders. In T. Ollendick & M. Hersen (Eds.), *Handbook of child psychopathology* (3rd ed., pp. 213-237). New York: Plenum Press.

Frick, P. J., & Loney, B. R. (1999). Outcomes of children and adolescents with oppositional defiant and analyses and cross-validation in a clinical sample. *Clinical Psychology Review, 13*, 319-340.

Frick, P. J., Stickle, T. R., Dandreaux, D. M., Farrell, J. M., & Kimonis, E. R. (2005). Callous-unemotional traits in predicting the severity and stability of conduct problems and delinquency. *Journal of Abnormal Child Psychology, 33*, 471-487.

Fromm, E. (1973). *The Anatomy of Human Destructiveness.* New York: Holt, Rinehart, and Winston.

Gallup Poll Online (October 6-8, 2003). Fear of crime/Fighting crime. Retrieved October 15, 2004 from http://www.galluppollonline.com

Garrison, C. Z., Waller, J. L., Cuffee, S. P., McKeown, R. E., Addy, C. L., & Jackson, K. L. (1997). Incidence of major depressive disorder and Dysthymia in young adolescents. *Journal of the American Academy of Child and Adolescent Psychiatry, 36,* 458-465.

Gendreau, P., Little, T., & Goggin, C. (1996). A meta-analysis of the predictors of adult offender recidivism: What works! *Criminology, 34,* 575-607.

Gjerde, P. F. (1995). Alternative pathways to chronic depressive symptoms in young adults: Gender differences in developmental trajectories. *Child Development, 66*(5), 1277-1300.

Gold, M. (1970). *Delinquent behavior in an American city.* Belmont, CA: Brooks/Cole Publishing Company.

Goldstein, A. L., Walton, M. A., Cunningham, R. M., Trowbridge, M. J., & Maio, R. F. (2007). Violence and substance use as risk factors for depressive symptoms among adolescents in an urban emergency department. *Journal of Adolescent Health, 40*, 276-279.

Goodyear, I., & Cooper, P. (1993). A community study of depression in adolescent girls: II. The clinical features of identified disorder. *British Journal of Psychiatry, 163*, 374-380.

Graham, S. (1992). "Most of the subjects were white and middle class": Trends in published research on African Americans in selected APA journals, 1979-1989. *American Psychologist, 47,* 629-639

Gurr, T. R. (1990). Historical trends in violent crime: A critical review of the evidence. In N.A. Weiner, M.A. Zahn, & R.J. Sagi (Eds.), *Violence: Patterns, causes, public policy* (pp. 15-23). Fort Worth, TX: Harcourt Brace.

Haller, J., & Kruk, M. R. (2006). Normal and abnormal aggression: Human disorders and novel laboratory models. *Neuroscience and Biobehavioral Reviews, 30,* 292-303.

Hammen, C., & Rudolph, K. D. (1996). Childhood depression. In E. J. Mash & R. A. Barkley (Eds.), *Child psychopathology* (pp. 153-195). New York: Guilford Press.

Hamparian, D. M., Schuster, R., Dinitz, S., & Conrad, J. (1978). *The violent few: A study of the dangerous juvenile offender.* Lexington, MA: Lexington Books.

Hanson, R. K., & Bussiere, M. T. (1998). Predicting relapse: A meta-analysis of sexual offender recidivism studies. *Journal of Consulting and Clinical Psychology, 66,* 348-362.

Hardin, J. W., & Hilbe, J. M. (2003). *Generalized estimating equations.* Norwell, MA: Chapman and Hall.

Harnish, J. D., Dodge, K. A., & Valente, E. (1995). Mother-child interaction quality as a partial mediator of the roles of maternal depressive symptomology and socioeconomic status in the development of child conduct disorders. *Child Development, 66,* 739-753.

Harrington, R., Fudge, H., Rutter, M., Pickles, A., & Hill, J. (1991). Adult outcomes of childhood and adolescent depression: II. Links with antisocial disorders. *Journal of the American Academy of Child & Adolescent Psychiatry, 30,* 434-439.

Harris, W. W., Lieberman, A. F., & Marans, S. (2007). In the best interests of society. *Journal of Child Psychology and Psychiatry, 48*(3/4), 392-411.

Heide, K. M. (1992). *Why kids kill parents: Child abuse and adolescent homicide.* Columbus, OH: Ohio State University Press.

Heide, K. M. (1995). Young killers: The challenge of juvenile homicide. Work in progress. *Lethal Violence: Proceedings of the 1995 Meeting of the Homicide Research Working Group.* Ottawa, Canada: Homicide Research Working Group.

Heide, K. M. (1999). *Young killers: The challenge of juvenile homicide.* Thousand Oaks, CA: Sage Publications.

Heide, K. M. (2004). Juvenile homicide encapsulated. In A. R. Roberts (Ed.), *Juvenile justice sourcebook* (pp. 423-464). New York: Oxford Press.

Heide, K. M., & Boots, D. P. (2003, November). *Parricide: An in-depth look at kids who kill parents and what happens to them.* Paper presented at the annual meeting of the American Society of Criminology, Denver, Colorado.

Heide, K. M., & Solomon, E. P. (2003). Treating today's juvenile homicide offenders. *Youth Violence and Juvenile Justice, 1*(1), 5-31.

Heitmeyer, W., & Hagan, J. (2003). *International handbook of violence research.* Norwell, MA: Kluwer Academic Press.

Henker, B., & Whalen, C. K. (1989). Hyperactivity and attention deficits. *American Psychologist, 44*, 216-244.

Hersen, M, & Ammerman, R. T. (2000). *Advanced abnormal child psychology.* Mahwah, NJ: Lawrence Erlbaum Associates.

Hindelang, M. J., Hirschi, T., & Weis, J. G. (1981). *Measuring delinquency.* Beverly Hills, CA: Sage Publishing.

Hinshaw, S. P., Lahey, B., & Hart, L. (1993). Issues of taxonomy and comorbidity in the development of conduct disorder. *Development and Psychopathology, 5*, 31-49.

Hirschfield, P., Maschi, T., White, H . R., Traub, L. G., & Loeber, R. (2006). Mental health and juvenile arrests: Criminality, criminalization, or compassion? *Criminology, 44*(3), 593-630.

Hollingshead, A. B. (1965). *Four factor index of social status.* New Haven, CT: Unpublished manuscript.

Howell, J. C., Krisberg, B., & Jones, M. (1995). Trends in juvenile crime and youth violence. In J. C Howell, B. Krisberg, J. D. Hawkins, & J. J. Wilson (Eds.), *A sourcebook: Serious, violent, & chronic juvenile offenders* (pp. 1-35). Thousand Oaks, CA: Sage Publications.

Huizinga, D., Esbensen, F., & Weiher, A. (1996). The impact of arrest on subsequent delinquent behavior. In R. Loeber, D. Huizinga, & R. P. Thornberry (Eds.), *Program of research on the causes and correlates of delinquency, Annual Report, 1995-1996* (pp. 82-101). Washington, DC: U.S. Department of Justice, Office of Justice Programs, Office of Juvenile Justice and Delinquency Prevention.

Huizinga, D., & Jakob-Chen, C. (1998). Contemporaneous co-occurrence of serious and violent juvenile offending and other problem behaviors. In R. Loeber and D. Farrington (Eds.), *Serious and violent juvenile offenders: Risk factors and successful interventions* (pp. 47-67). Thousand Oaks, CA: Sage Publications.

Huizinga, D., Loeber, R., Thornberry, T. P., & Cothern, L. (2000). Co-occurrence of delinquency and other problem behaviors. *Juvenile Justice Bulletin*. Washington, DC: U.S. Department of Justice.

Ialongo, N., Edelsohn, G., Werthamer-Larsson, L., Crockett, L., & Kellam, S. (1995). The significance of self-reported anxious symptoms in first grade children: Prediction to anxious symptoms and adaptive functioning in fifth grade. *Journal of Child Psychology and Psychiatry and Allied Disciplines, 36*, 427-437.

Jeglum-Bartusch, D., Lynam, D., Moffitt, T. E., & Silva, P. A. (1997). Is age important? Testing general versus developmental theories of antisocial behavior. *Criminology, 35*, 13-47.

Jenson, J. M., & Howard, M. O. (1999). *Youth violence: Current research and recent practice innovations.* Washington, DC: National Association of Social Workers Press.

Kagan, J., Reznick, J. S., & Snidman, N. (1988). Biological bases of childhood shyness. *Science, 240,* 167-171.

Kasen, S., Cohen, P., Skodol, A. E., Johnson, J. G., Smailes, E., & Brook, J. S. (2001). Childhood depression and adult personality disorder. *Archives of General Psychiatry, 58*, 231-236.

Kashani, J. H., Dahlmeier, J. M., Borduin, C. M., Soltys, S., & Reid, J. C. (1995). Characteristics of anger expression in depressed children. *Journal of the American Academy of Child and Adolescent Psychiatry, 34*, 322-326.

Kellam, S. G., Ensminger, M. E., & Simon, M. B. (1980). Mental health in first grade and teenage drug, alcohol, and cigarette use. *Drug and Alcohol Dependency, 5*, 273-304.

Kempf, K. (1988). Crime severity and criminal career progression. *Journal of Criminal Law and Criminology, 79*, 201-216.

Kempf-Leonard, K., Tracy, P. E., & Howell, J. C. (2001). Serious, violent, and chronic juvenile offenders: The relationship of delinquency career types to adult criminality. *Justice Quarterly, 18*(3), 449-478.

Kessler, R. C., & Walters, E. E. (1998). Epidemiology of DSM-III-R major depression and minor depression among adolescents and young adults in the National Comorbidity Survey. *Depression and Anxiety, 7*, 3-14.

Kilgore, K., Snyder, J., & Lentz, C. (2000). The contribution of parental discipline, parental monitoring, and school risk to early-onset conduct problems in African American boys and girls. *Developmental Psychology, 36*, 835-845.

King, G., & Zeng, L. (2001). Explaining rare events in international relations. *International Organization, 55*(3), 693-715.

Kiser, L. J. (2007). Protecting children from the dangers of urban poverty. *Clinical Psychology Review, 27*, 211-225.

Klein, D. N., Lewinsohn, P. M., & Seeley, J. R. (1996). Hypomanic personality traits in a community sample of adolescents. *Journal of Affective Disorders, 38*, 135-143.

Klein, M. W. (1995). *The American street gang.* New York: Oxford University Press.

Kline, F., M., & Silver, L. B. (2004). *The educator's guide to mental health issues in the classroom.* Baltimore, MD: Paul H. Brookes Publishing.

Knox, M., King, C., Hanna, G.L., Logan, D., & Ghaziuddin, N. (2000). Aggressive behavior in clinically depressed adolescents. *Journal of the American Academy of Child and Adolescent Psychiatry, 29*, 611-618.

Kovacs, M. (1996). Presentation and course of major depressive disorder during childhood and later years of the life span. *Journal of the American Academy of Child and Adolescent Psychiatry, 35*, 705-715.

Kovacs, M., Akiskal, H. S., Gatsonis, C., & Parrone, P. L. (1994). Childhood-onset dysthymic disorder: Clinical features and prospective naturalistic outcome. *Archives of General Psychiatry, 51*, 365-374.

Kovacs, M., Feinberg, T. L., Crouse-Novak, M. A., Paulauskas, S. L., & Finkelstein, R. (1984). Depressive disorders in childhood. I. A longitudinal prospective study of characteristics and recovery. *Archives of General Psychiatry, 41*, 229-237.

Kovacs, M., & Gatsonis, C. (1994). Secular trends in age at onset of major depressive disorder in a clinical sample of children. *Journal of Psychiatric Research, 28*, 319-329.

Kovacs, M., Obrosky, D. S., Gastonis, C., & Richards, C. (1997). First-episode major depressive and Dysthymic disorder in childhood: Clinical and sociodemographic factors in recovery. *Journal of American Academy of Child and Adolescent Psychiatry, 36*, 777-784.

Koyanagi, C. (1999). *Making sense of Medicaid for children with serious emotional disturbance.* Washington, DC: Bazelon Center for Mental Health Law.

Krol, N. P., De Bruyn, E. E . J., Coolen, J. C., & van Aarle, E. J. M.. (2006). From CBCL to *DSM*: A comparison of two methods to screen for *DSM-IV* diagnoses using CBCL data. *Journal of Clinical Child and Adolescent Psychology, 35*(1), 127-135.

Kurtz, L. (Ed.) (1999). *Encyclopedia of violence, peace, conflict.* New York: Academic Press.

Lahey, B. B., Applegate, B., McBurnett, K., Biederman, J., Greenhill, L., Hynd, G. W., Barkley, R. A., Newcorn, J., Jensen, P., Richters, J., Garfinkel, B., Kerdyk, L., Frick, P. J., Ollendick, T., Perez, D., Hart, E. L., Waldman, I., & Shaffer, D. (1994). DSM-IV field trials for attention deficit/hyperactivity disorder in children and adolescents. *Journal of the American Academy of Child and Adolescent Psychiatry, 151*, 1673-1685.

Lahey, B. B., & Loeber, R. (1994). Framework for a developmental model of oppositional defiant disorder and conduct disorder. In D. K. Routh (Ed.), *Disruptive behavior disorders in childhood* (pp. 139-180). New York: Plenum Press.

Lahey, B. B., Loeber, R., Hart, E. L., Frick, P., Applegate, B., Zhang, Q., Green, S. M., & Russo, M. F. (1995). Four-year longitudinal study of Conduct Disorder in boys: Patterns and predictors of persistence. *Journal of Abnormal Psychology, 104*, 83-93.

Lahey, B. B., Miller, T. L., Gordon, R. A., & Riley, A. W. (1999). Developmental epidemiology of the disruptive behavior disorders. In H.C. Quay and A. Hogan (Eds.), *Handbook of Disruptive Behavior Disorders* (pp. 23-48). New York: Plenum Press.

Lahey, B. B., & Waldman, I. D. (2005). A developmental model of the propensity to offend during childhood and adolescence. In D. P. Farrington (Ed.), *Integrated developmental & life-course theories of offending: Advances in Criminological Theory* (Vol. 14, pp. 15-50). New Brunswick, NJ: Transaction Publishers.

Landy, S., & Peters, R. D. (1991, February). Understanding and treating the hyperaggressive toddler. *Zero to Three,* 22-31.

Lane, R. (1997). *Murder in America: A history.* Columbus, OH: Ohio State University Press.

Langbehn, D. R., Cadoret, R. J., Yates, W. R., Troughton, E. P., & Stewart, M. A. (1998). Distinct contributions of conduct and oppositional defiant symptoms to adult antisocial behavior. *Archives of General Psychiatry, 55,* 821-829.

Laub, J. H., Nagin, D. S., & Sampson, R. J. (1998). Good marriages and trajectories of change in criminal offending. *American Sociological Review, 63,* 225-238.

Laub, J. H., & Sampson, R. J. (2003). *Shared beginnings, divergent lives: Delinquent boys to age 70.* Cambridge, MA: Harvard University Press.

Leaf, P. J., Alegria, M., Cohen, P., Goodman, S. H., Horowitz, S., Hoven, C. W., Narrow, W. E., Vaden-Kiernan, M., & Regier, D. A. (1996). Mental health service use in the community and schools: Results from the four-community MECA study. *Journal of the American Academy of Child and Adolescent Psychiatry, 35,* 889-896.

Le Blanc, M., & Loeber, R. (1998). Developmental criminology updated. In M. Tonry (Ed.), *Crime and Justice: A Review of Research* (Vol. 23, pp. 115-198). Chicago: University of Chicago Press.

Lee, B. J. (1987). Multidisciplinary evaluation of preschool children and ts demography in a military psychiatric clinic. *Journal of the American Academy of Child and Adolescent Psychiatry, 26,* 313-316.

Lemert, E. M. (1951). *Social pathology.* New York: McGraw-Hill.

Lemert, E. M. (1967). The juvenile court: Quest and realities in the President's Commission on Law Enforcement and Administration of Justice. *Task Force Report: Juvenile delinquency and youth crime.* Washington, DC: U.S. Government Printing Office.

Lemery, K. S., Essex, M. J., & Smider, N. A. (2002). Revealing the relationship between temperament and behavioral problems by eliminating measurement confounding: Expert ratings and factor analysis. *Child Development, 73*, 867-882.

Lewinsohn, P. M., Hops, H., Roberts, R. E., Seeley, J. R., & Andrews, J. A. (1993). Adolescent psychopathology: I. Prevalence and incidence of depression and other DSM-III-R disorders in high school students. *Journal of Abnormal Psychology, 102*, 133-144.

Li, S. T., Nussbaum, K. M., & Richards, M. H. (2007). Risk and protective factors for urban African-American youth. *American Journal of Community Psychology, 39*, 21-35.

Lien, L., Haavet, O.R., Thoresen, M., Heyerdahl, S., & Bjertness, E. (2007). Mental health problems, negative life events, perceived pressure and the frequency of acute infections among adolescents – Results from a cross-sectional, multicultural, population-based study. *Acta Paediatrica, 96*(2), 301-306.

Linehan, M. M., Heard, H. L., & Armstrong, H. E. (1993). Naturalistic follow-up of a behavioral treatment for chronically parasuicidal borderline patients. *Archives of General Psychiatry, 50*, 971-974.

Link, B. G., Cullen, F. T., Struening, E., Shrout, P., & Dohrenwend, B. P. (1989). A modified labeling theory approach in the area of the mental disorders: An empirical assessment. *American Sociological Review, 54*, 400-423.

Link, B. G., Phelan, J. C., Bresnahan, M., Stueve, A., & Pescosolido, B. A. (1999). Public conceptions of mental illness: Labels, causes, dangerousness, and social distance. *American Journal of Public Health, 89*, 1328-1333.

Link, B. G., & Steuve, C (1994). Psychotic symptoms and the violent/illegal behavior of mental patients compared to community controls. In J. Monahan & H.J. Steadman (Eds.), *Violence and Mental Disorder: Developments in Risk Assessment* (pp. 137-159). Chicago: University of Chicago Press.

Loeber, R. (1982). The stability of antisocial and delinquent behavior: A review. *Child Development, 53*, 1431-1446.

Loeber, R. (1991). Antisocial behavior: More enduring than changeable? *Journal of the American Academy of Child and Adolescent Psychiatry, 31*, 393-397.

Loeber, R. (2004). *Delinquency prevention in a mental health context.* Utrecht, Netherlands: Trimbos Institute.

Loeber, R., Burke, J. D., & Lahey, B. B. (2002). What are adolescent antecedents to antisocial personality disorder? *Criminal Behaviour and Mental Health, 12,* 24-36.

Loeber, R., Burke, J. D., Lahey, B. B., Winters, A., & Zera, M. (2000). Oppositional defiant and conduct disorder: A review of the past 10 years, Part I. *Journal of the American Academy of Child and Adolescent Psychiatry, 39*(12), 1-17.

Loeber, R. & Dishion, T. J. (1983). Early predictors of male delinquency: A review. *Psychological Bulletin, 94,* 68-99.

Loeber, R., & Farrington, D. P. (Eds.) (1998). *Serious and violent juvenile offenders: Risk factors and successful interventions.* Thousand Oaks, CA: Sage Publications.

Loeber, R., & Farrington, D. P. (2000). Young children who commit crime: Epidemiology, developmental origins, risk factors, early interventions, and policy implications. *Development and Psychopathology, 12*(4), 737-762.

Loeber, R., & Farrington, D. P. (2001). *Child delinquents: Development, intervention and service needs.* Thousand Oaks, CA: Sage Publications.

Loeber, R., Farrington, D. P., Stouthamer-Loeber, M., Moffitt, T. E., Caspi, A., White, H. R., Wei, E. H., & Beyers, J. M. (2003). The development of male offending: Key findings from fourteen year of the Pittsburgh Youth Study. In T.P. Thornberry and M.D. Krohn (Eds.), *Taking stock of delinquency: An overview of findings from contemporary longitudinal studies* (pp. 93-136). New York: Kluwer Academic/Plenum Publishers.

Loeber, R., Farrington, D. P., Stouthamer-Loeber, M., & Van Kammen, W. B. (1998). *Antisocial behavior and mental health problems: Explanatory factors in childhood and adolescence.* Mahwah, NJ: Lawrence Erlbaum Associates.

Loeber, R., Farrington, D. P., & Waschbusch, D. A. (2001). Serious and violent juvenile offenders. In R. Loeber & D. P. Farrington (Eds.), *Serious & violent juvenile offenders: Risk factors and successful interventions* (pp. 13-29). Thousand Oaks, CA: Sage Publishers.

Loeber, R., Green, S. M., Lahey, B. B., Christ, M. A. G., & Frick, P. J. (1992). Developmental sequences in the age of onset of disruptive child behaviors. *Journal of Child and Family Studies, 1*, 21-41.

Loeber, R., Green, S. M., Lahey, B. B., & Kalb, L. (2000). Physical fighting in childhood as a risk factor for later mental health problems. *Journal of the American Academy of Child and Adolescent Psychiatry, 39*, 421-428.

Loeber, R., & Hay, D. F. (1994). Developmental approaches to aggression and conduct problems. In M.L. Rutter & D.H. Hay (Eds.), *Development through life: A handbook for clinicians* (pp. 488-515). Oxford: Blackwell.

Loeber, R. & Keenan, K. (1994). The interaction between conduct disorder and its comorbid conditions: Effects of age and gender. *Clinical Psychology Review, 14*, 497-523.

Loeber, R., Lahey, B. B., & Thomas, C. (1991). Diagnostic conundrum of oppositional defiant disorder and conduct disorder. *Journal of Abnormal Psychology, 100*, 379-390.

Loeber, R., & Le Blanc, M. (1990). Toward a developmental criminology. In M. Tonry & N. Morris (Eds.), *Crime and justice: An annual review of research* (Vol. 12, pp. 375-473). Chicago: University of Chicago Press.

Loeber, R., Pardini, D., Homish, D. L., Wei, E. H., Crawford, A. M., Farrington, D. P., Stouthamer-Loeber, M., Creemers, J., Koehler, S. A., & Rosenfeld, R. (2005). The prediction of violence and homicide in young men. *Journal of Consulting and Clinical Psychology, 73*(6), 1074-1088.

Loeber, R., Russo, M. F., Stouthamer-Loeber, M., & Lahey, B. B. (1994). Internalizing problems and their relation to the development of disruptive behaviors in adolescence. *Journal of Research on Adolescence, 4*, 61-637.

Loeber, R., & Schmaling, K. B. (1985). The utility of differentiating between mixed and pure forms of antisocial child behavior. *Journal of Abnormal Child Psychology, 13*, 315-335.

Loeber, R., Stouthamer-Loeber, M., & Green, S. M. (1991). Age at onset of problem behavior in boys, and later disruptive and delinquent behavior. *Criminal Behavior and Mental Health, 1*, 229-246.

Loeber, R., Stouthamer-Loeber, M., Farrington, D. P., Lahey, B. B., Kennan, K., & White, H. R. (2002). Editorial introduction. Three longitudinal studies of children's development in Pittsburgh. The Developmental Trends Study, the Pittsburgh Youth Study, and the Pittsburgh Girls Study. *Criminal Behaviour and Mental Health, 12*, 1-23.

Loeber, R., Stouthamer-Loeber, M., & White, H. R. (1999). Developmental aspects of delinquency and internalizing problems and their association with persistent juvenile substance use between ages 7 and 18. *Journal of Clinical Child Psychology, 28*(3), 322-332.

Lynam, D. R., Caspi, A., Moffitt, T. E., Loeber, R., & Stouthamer-Loeber, M. (2007). Longitudinal evidence that psychopathy scores in early adolescence predict adult psychopathy. *Journal of Abnormal Psychology, 116*(1), 155-165.

MacKinnon-Lewis, C., Kaufman, M. C., & Frabutt, J. M. (2002). Juvenile justice and mental health: Youth and families in the middle. *Aggression and Violent Behavior, 7*, 353-363.

Marcus, S. C., Olfson, M., Pincus, H. A., Shear, M. K., & Zarin, D. A. (1997). Self-reported anxiety, general medical conditions, and disability bed days. *American Journal of Psychiatry, 154*, 1766-1768.

Marzuk, P. M. (1996). Violence, crime and mental illness. How strong a link? *Archives of General Psychiatry, 53*, 481-486.

Mash, E. J., & Wolfe, D. A. (2005). *Abnormal child psychology* (3rd ed.). Belmont, CA: Wadsworth/Thomson.

Mazerolle, P., Brame, R., Paternoster, R., Piquero, A., & Dean, C. (2000). Onset age, persistence, and offending versatility. Comparisons across gender. *Criminology, 38*, 1143-1172.

Maughan, B., & Rutter, M. (1998). Continuities and discontinuities in antisocial behavior from childhood to adult life. In T. H. Ollendick & R. J. Prinz (Eds.), *Advances in clinical child psychology* (Vol. 20, pp. 1-47). New York: Plenum Press.

McElhaney, S. J., Russell, M., & Barton, H. A. (1993). *Children's mental health and their ability to learn.* Washington, DC: National Health/Education Consortium.

McGee, R., & Williams, S. (1988). A longitudinal study of depression in nine year old children. *Journal of the American Academy of Child and Adolescent Psychiatry, 27,* 12-20.

McGrath, R.D. (1984). *Gunfighters, highwaymen, and vigilantes: Violence on the frontier.* Berkeley: University of California.

McMahon, R. J., & Forehand, R. (2003). *Helping the noncompliant child: Family-based treatment for oppositional behavior* (2nd ed.). New York: Guilford Press.

Meadows, R.J., & Kuehnel, J.M. (2005). *Evil minds: Understanding and responding to violent predators.* Upper Saddle River, NJ: Pearson Prentice Hall.

Mertler, C. A., & Vannatta, R. A. (2005). *Advanced and multivariate statistical methods: Practical application and interpretation* (3rd ed.). Glendale, CA: Pyrczak Publishing.

Miech, R. A., Caspi, A., Moffitt, T. E., Wright, B. R. E., & Silva, P. A. (1999). Low socioeconomic status and mental disorders: A longitudinal study of selection and causation during young adulthood. *American Journal of Sociology, 104,* 1096-1131.

Miller, J. E. (2005). *The Chicago guide to writing about multivariate analysis.* Chicago: University of Chicago Press.

Millon, T. (1996). *Disorders of personality: DSM-IV and beyond.* New York: John Wiley & Sons.

Mitchell, J., McCauley, E., Burke, P.M., & Moss, S.J. (1988). Phenomenology of depression in children and adolescents. *Journal of the American Academy of Child and Adolescent Psychiatry, 27,* 12-20.

Moffitt, T. E. (1990). Juvenile delinquency and attention deficit disorder: Boys' developmental trajectories from age 13 to age 15. *Child Development, 61,* 893-910.

Moffitt, T. E. (1993). Adolescence-limited and life-course-persistent antisocial behavior: A developmental taxonomy. *Psychological Review, 100,* 674-701.

Moffitt, T. E. (2001). Adolescence-limited and life-course persistent antisocial behavior. In A. Piquero & P. Mazerolle (Eds.), *Life-course criminology: Contemporary and classic readings.* Stamford, CT: Wadsworth/Thomson Learning.

Moffitt, T. E., Caspi, A., Dickson, N., Silva, P., & Stanton, W. (1996). Childhood-onset versus adolescent-onset antisocial conduct problems in males: Natural history from ages 3 to 18. *Development and Psychology, 8*, 399-424.

Moffitt, T. E., Caspi, A., Harrington, H., & Milne, B. J. (2002). Males on the life-course-persistent and adolescence-limited antisocial pathways: Follow-up at age 26 years. *Development and Psychopathology, 14*, 179-207.

Moffitt, T. E., Caspi, A., Rutter, M., & Silva, P. A. (2001). *Sex differences in antisocial behaviour: Conduct disorder, delinquency, and violence in the Dunedin Longitudinal Study.* New York: Cambridge University Press.

Moffitt, T. E., Lynam, D., & Silva, P. A. (1994). Neuropsychological tests predict persistent male delinquency. *Criminology, 32*, 101-124.

Moffitt, T. E., & Silva, P.A. (1988). Self-reported delinquency, neuro-psychological deficit, and history of attention deficit disorder. *Journal of Abnormal Child Psychology, 16*, 553-569.

Moone, J. (1994). *Juvenile victimization: 1987-1992. Fact sheet #17.* Washington, DC: U.S. Department of Justice, Office of Juvenile Justice and Delinquency Prevention.

Monahan, J. (1992). Mental disorder and violent behavior: Perceptions and evidence. *American Psychologist, 47,* 511-521.

Mullen, P. E. (1997). A reassessment of the link between mental disorder and violent behaviour, and its implications for clinical practice. *Australian and New Zealand Journal of Psychiatry, 31*, 3-11.

Mullen, P. E., Burgess, P., Wallace, C., Palmer, S., & Ruschena, D. (2000). Community care and criminal offending in schizophrenia. *Lancet, 355*, 614-617.

Mulvey, E. P. (1994). Assessing the evidence of a link between mental illness and violence. *Hospital and Community Psychiatry, 45*, 663-668.

Nagin, D. S., & Tremblay, R. E. (1999). Trajectories of boys' physical aggression, oppositional, and hyperactivity on the path to physically violent and nonviolent juvenile delinquency. *Child Development, 70,* 1181-1196.

National Institute of Mental Health (NIMH) (2001). *Blueprint of change: Research on child and adolescent mental health. Report of the National Advisory Mental Health Council's Workgroup on Child and Adolescent Mental Health Intervention Development and Deployment.* Washington, DC: U.S. Government Printing Office.

Norusis, M. J. (1998). *SPSS 8.0: Guide to data analysis.* Upper Saddle River, NJ: Prentice Hall.

Nunnally, J. (1961). *Popular conceptions of mental health.* New York: Holt, Rinehart and Winston.

Offord, D. R., Boyle, M. C., & Racine, Y. A., (1991). The epidemiology of antisocial behavior in childhood and adolescence. In D. J. Pepler & K. H., Rubin (Eds.), *The development and treatment of childhood aggression* (pp. 31-54). Hillsdale, NJ: Lawrence Erlbaum Associates.

Offord, D. R., Lipman, E. L., & Duku, E. K. (2001). Epidemiology of problem behavior up to age 12 years. In R. Loeber & D. P. Farrington (Eds.), *Child delinquents: Development, intervention, and service needs* (pp. 95-116). Thousand Oaks, CA: Sage Publications.

Oldehinkel, A. J., Hartman, C. A., de Winter, A. F., Veenstra, R., & Ormel, J. (2004). Temperament profiles associated with internalizing and externalizing problems in preadolescence. *Development and Psychopathology, 16,* 421-440.

Oldehinkel, A. J., Veenstra, R., Ormel, J., de Winter, A. F., & Verhulst, F. C. (2006). Temperament, parenting, and depressing symptoms in a population sample of preadolescents. *Journal of Child Psychology and Psychiatry, 47*(7). 684-695.

Olvera, R. L. (2002). Intermittent explosive disorder: Epidemiology, diagnosis, and management. *CNS Drugs, 16,* 517-526.

Otto, R. K., Greenstein, J. J., Johnson, M. K., & Friedman, R. M. (1992). Prevalence of mental disorders among youth in the juvenile justice system. In J. J. Cocozza (Ed.), *Responding to the mental health needs of youth in the juvenile justice system* (pp. 7-28). Seattle, WA: National Coalition for the Mentally Ill in the Criminal Justice System.

Patel, V., Flisher, A. J., Hetrick, S., & McGorry, P. (2007). Mental health of young people: A global public-health challenge. *The Lancet, 369*, 1302-1313.

Patterson, G. R. (1982). *Coercive family processes.* Eugene, OR: Castalia Press.

Patterson, G. R. (1986). Performance models for antisocial boys. *American Psychologist, 41*, 432-444.

Patterson, G. R., DeBaryshe, B. D., & Ramsey, E. (1989). A developmental perspective on antisocial behavior. *American Psychologist, 44*(2), 329-335.

Phares, V., & Danforth, J. S. (1994). Adolescents', parents', and teachers' distress over adolescents' behavior. *Journal of Abnormal Child Psychology, 22*(6), 721-733.

Phelan, J. C., & Link, B. G. (1998). The growing belief that people with mental illnesses are violent: The role of the dangerousness criterion for civil commitment. *Social Psychiatry and Psychiatric Epidemiology, 33*, S7-S12.

Piquero, A. R., Brame, R., Mazerolle, P., & Haapanen, R. (2002). Crime in emerging adulthood. *Criminology, 40*, 137-170.

Piquero, A., MacDonald, J., Dobrin, A., Daigle, L. E., & Cullen, F. T. (2005). Self-control, violent offending, and homicide victimization: Assessing the general theory of crime. *Journal of Quantitative Criminology, 21*(1), 55-71.

Piquero, A. R., & Mazerolle, P. (Eds.). (2001). *Life-course criminology: Contemporary and classic readings.* Belmont, CA: Wadsworth/Thomson Learning.

Piquero, A. R., & Moffitt, T. E. (2005). Explaining the facts of crime: How the developmental taxonomy replies to Farrington's invitation. In D. P. Farrington (Ed.), *Integrated developmental & life-course theories of offending: Advances in Criminology Theory* (Vol. 14, pp. 51-72). New Brunswick, NJ: Transaction Publishers.

Pliszka, S.R. (1998). Comorbidity of attention deficit/hyperactivity disorder with psychiatric disorder: An overview. *Journal of Clinical Psychiatry, 59*, 50-58.

Popper, S. D, Ross, S., & Jennings, K. D. (2000). Development and psychopathology. In M. Hersen and R.T. Ammerman (Eds.), *Advanced abnormal child psychology,* (pp. 47-56). Mahwah, NJ: Lawrence Erlbaum Associates.

Pottic, K. J., Hsieh, D. K., Kirk, S. A., & Tian, X. (2007). Judging mental disorder in youths: Effects of client, clinician, and contextual diffeences. *Journal of Consulting and Clinical Psychology, 75*(1), 1-8.

Puis-Antich, J. (1982). Major depression and conduct disorder in prepuberty. *Journal of the American Academy of Child and Adolescent Psychiatry, 21*, 118-128.

Puig-Antich, J., Goetz, D., Davies, M., Kaplan, T., Davies, S., Ostrow, L., Asnis, L., Twomey, J., Iyengar, S., & Ryan, N. D. (1989). A controlled family history study of prepubertal major depressive disorders. *Archives of General Psychiatry, 46*, 406-418.

Puig-Antich, J., Lukens, E., Davies, M., Goetz, D., Brennan-Quattrock, J., Todak, G. (1985). Psychosocial functioning in prepubertal major depressive disorders. *Archives of General Psychiatry, 42*, 500-507.

Rabian, B., & Silverman, W. K. (2000). Anxiety disorders. In M. Hersen & R. T. Ammerman (Eds.), *Advanced abnormal child psychology* (2nd ed., pp. 271-289). Mahwah, NJ: Lawrence Erlbaum Associates.

Radke-Yarrow, M., Campbell, J. D., & Burton, R. V. (1968). *Childbearing: An inquiry into research and methods.* San Francisco: Jossey-Bass.

Rapport, M. D., & Chung, K. (2000). Attention deficit hyperactivity disorder. In M. Hersen and R.T. Ammerman (Eds.), *Advanced abnormal child psychology* (pp. 413-440). Mahwah, NJ: Lawrence Erlbaum Associates.

Regier, D. A., Kaelber, C. T., Rae, D. S., Farmer, M. E., Knauper, B., Kessler, R. C., & Norquist, G. S. (1998). Limitations of diagnostic criteria and assessment instruments for mental disorders: Implications for research and policy. *Archives of General Psychiatry, 55*, 109-115.

Reid, J. B. (1993). Prevention of conduct disorder before and after school entry: Relating interventions to developmental findings. *Development and Psychopathology, 5,* 243-262.

Reidel, M., & Welsh, W. (2002). *Criminal violence- Patterns, causes, and prevention.* Los Angeles: Roxbury.

Reiss, A. J., & Roth, J. A. (eds.) (1993). *Understanding and preventing violence.* Washington, DC: National Academy Press.

Renk, K., & Phares, V. (2004). Cross-informant ratings of social competence in children and adolescents. *Clinical Psychology Review, 24,* 239-254.

Rescorla, L, Achenbach, T. M., Ivanova, M. Y., Dumenci, L., Almqvist, F., Bilenberg, N., Bird, H., Broberg, A., Dobrean, A., Dopfner, M., Erol, N., Forns, M., Hannesdottir, H., Kanbayashi, Y., Lambert, M. C., Leung, P., Minaei, A., Malutu, M. S., Novik, T. S., Oh, K. J., Roussos, A., Sawyer, M., Simsek, Z., Steinhausen, H. C., Weintraub, S., Metzke, C. W., Wolanczyk, T., Zilber, N., Zukauskiene, R., & Verhulst, F. (2007). Epidemiological comparisons of problems and positive qualities reported by adolescents in 24 countries. *Journal of Consulting and Clinical Psychology, 75*(2), 351-358.

Richman, N., & Graham, P. (1975). A behavioral screening questionnaire for use with three-year old children: Preliminary findings. *Journal of Child Psychology and Psychiatry, 16,* 277-287.

Richman, N., Stevenson, J., & Graham, P. (1982). *Preschool to school: A behavioural study.* New York: Academic Press.

Robins, L., & Helzer, J. E. (1994). The half-life of a structured interview: The NIMH Diagnostic Interview Schedule (DIS). *International Journal of Methods in Psychiatry Research, 4,* 95-102.

Ross, D. M., & Ross, S. A. (1982). *Hyperactivity: Current issues, research, and theory.* New York: Wiley.

Routh, D. K. (Ed.) (1994). *Disruptive behavior disorders in childhood.* New York: Plenum Press.

Rudolph, K. D., Hammen, C., & Daley, S. E. (2006). Mood disorders. In D. A. Wolfe & E. J. Mash (Eds.), *Behavioral and emotional disorders in adolescents: Nature, assessment, and treatment* (pp. 300-342). New York: Guilford Press.

Russo, M. F., & Beidel, D. C. (1994). Co-morbidity of childhood anxiety and externalizing disorders: Prevalence, associated characteristics, and validation issues. *Clinical Psychology Review, 14*, 199-221.

Rutter, M. L. (1986). Child psychiatry: The interface between clinical and developmental research. *Psychological Medicine, 16*, 151-169.

Ryan, N. D., Puig-Antich, J., Ambrosini, P., Rabinovich, J., Robinson, D., Nelson, B., Iyengar, S., Twomey, J. (1987). The clinical picture of major depression in children and adolescents. *Archives of General Psychiatry, 44*, 854-861.

Safer, D., & Allen, R. (1976). *Hyperactive children: Diagnosis and management.* Baltimore: University Park Press.

Sampson, R. J., & Laub, J. H. (1990). Crime and deviance over the life course: The salience of adult social bonds. *American Sociological Review, 55,* 609-627.

Sampson, R. J., & Laub, J. H. (1993). *Crime in the making: Pathways and turning points through life.* Cambridge, MA: Harvard University Press.

Sampson, R. J., & Laub, J. H. (1994). Urban poverty and the family context of delinquency: A new look at structure and process in a classic study. *Child Development, 55*, 523-540.

Sampson, R. J., & Laub, J. H. (2001). Crime and deviance in the Life Course. In A. Piquero & P. Mazerolle (Eds.), *Life-Course criminology: Contemporary and classic readings* (pp. 21-42). Belmont, CA: Wadsworth/Thomson Learning.

Satterfield, J. H., Swanson, J., Schell, A., & Lee, F. (1994). Prediction of antisocial behavior in attention-deficit hyperactivity disorder boys from aggression/defiance scores. *Journal of the American Academy of Child and Adolescent Psychiatry, 33*, 185-191.

Saunders, B. E. (2003). Understanding children exposed to violence: Toward an integration of overlapping fields. *Journal of Interpersonal Violence, 18*, 356-376.

Shorr, L. (1997). *Common purpose: Strengthening families and neighborhood to rebuild America.* New York: Anchor Book Place.

Simons, R. L., Johnson, C., Conger, R. D., & Elder, G. (1998). A test of latent trait versus life course perspectives on the stability of adolescent antisocial behavior. *Criminology, 36,* 217-243.

Skogan, W. G. (1989). Social change and the future of violent crime. In
    T. R. Gurr (Ed.), *Violence in America: Vol. 1. The history of crime*
    (pp. 235-250). Newbury Park, CA: Sage Publications.
Snyder, H. N. (1988). *Court careers of juvenile offenders.* Washington,
    DC: U.S. Department of Justice, Office of Juvenile Justice and
    Delinquency Prevention.
Snyder, H. N. (2003). *Juvenile arrests 2001.* Washington, DC: U.S.
    Department of Justice, Office of Juvenile Justice and Delinquency
    Prevention.
Spergel, I. A. (1990). Youth gangs: Continuity and change. In M.
    Tonry and N. Morris (Eds.), *Crime and justice: A review of
    research* (Vol. 12, pp. 171-275). Chicago: University of Chicago
    Press.
Spitzer, R. L., Williams, J. B. W., & Skodol, A. E. (1980). DSM-III:
    The major achievements and an overview. *American Journal of
    Psychiatry, 137,* 151-164.
Sprafkin, J., & Gadow, K. D. (1996). *Early Childhood Inventories
    Manual.* Stony Brook, NY: Checkmate Plus.
Stark, K. D., Bronik, M. D., Wong, S., Wells, G., & Ostrander, R.
    (2000). Depressive disorders. In M. Hersen and R.T. Ammerman
    (Eds.), *Advanced abnormal child psychology* (pp. 291-326).
    Mahwah, NJ: Lawrence Erlbaum Associates.
Stevens, J. (1992). *Applied multivariate statistics for the social
    sciences. (2nd ed.).* Hillsdale, NJ: Lawrence Erlbaum Associates.
Stouthamer-Loeber, M. (1993). Optimizing data quality of individual
    and community sources in longitudinal research. In D. P.
    Farrington, R. J. Sampson, & P. O. Wikstrom (Eds.), *Integrating
    individual and ecological aspects of crime* (pp. 259-277).
    Stockholm, Sweden: National Council for Crime Prevention.
Stouthamer-Loeber, M., & Van Kammen, W. B. (1995). *Data
    collection and management: A practical guide.* Applied Social
    Research Methods Series. Thousand Oaks, CA: Sage Publications.
Stouthamer-Loeber, M. (1993). Optimizing data quality of individual
    and community sources in longitudinal research. In D. P.
    Farrington, R. J. Sampson, & P.O. Wikstrom (Eds.), *Integrating
    individual and ecological aspects of crime* (pp. 259-277).
    Stockholm, Sweden: National Council for Crime Prevention.
Strasburg, P. (1978). *Violent delinquents.* New York: Monarch Press.

Strauss, C. C., Lease, C. A., Last, C. G., & Francis, G. (1988). Overanxious disorder: An examination of developmental differences. *Journal of Abnormal Child Psychology, 16*, 433-443.

Swanson, J. W., Holzer, C. E., Ganju, V. K., & Jono, R. T. (1990). Violence and psychiatric disorder in the community: Evidence from the epidemiological catchment area surveys. *Hospital and Community Psychiatry, 41*, 761-770.

Szatmari, P. (1992). The epidemiology of attention-deficit hyperactivity disorders. *Child and Adolescent Psychiatry Clinics of North America, 1*, 361-372.

Tarnowski, K. J., & Blechman, E. A. (1991). Disadvantaged children and families. *Journal of Clinical Child Psychology, 20*, 338-339.

Taylor, P. J., Garety, P., Buchanan, A., Reed, A., Wessely, S., Ray, K., Dunn, G., & Grubin, D. (1994). Delusions and violence. In J. Monahan & H.J. Steadman (Eds.), *Violence and mental disorder: Developments in risk assessment* (pp. 161-182). Chicago: University of Chicago Press.

Teplin, L. A. (2001). *Assessing alcohol, drug,, and mental disorders in juvenile detainees*. Office of Juvenile Justice and Delinquency Fact Sheet #02. Washington, DC: U.S. Department of Justice.

Tolan, P. H., & Gorman-Smith, D. (1998). Development of serious and violent offending careers. In R. Loeber & D. P. Farrington (Eds.), *Serious and violent juvenile offenders: Risk factors and successful interventions* (pp. 68-85). Thousand Oaks, CA: Sage Publications.

Thornberry, T. P. (1998). Membership in youth gangs and involvement in serious violent offending. In R. Loeber & D. P. Farrington (Eds.), *Serious and violent juvenile offenders: Risk factors and successful interventions* (pp. 147-166). Thousand Oaks, CA: Sage Publications.

Thornberry, T. P., Huizinga, D., & Loeber, R. (1995). The prevention of serious delinquency and violence: Implications from the Program of Research on the Causes and Correlates of Delinquency. In J. C. Howell, B. Krisberg, J. D. Hawkins, & J. J. Wilson (Eds.), *Sourcebook on serious, violent, and chronic juvenile offenders* (pp. 213-237). Thousand Oaks, CA: Sage Publications.

Thornberry, T., & Krohn, M. (2000). The self-report method for measuring delinquency and crime. In D. Duffee (Ed.), *Measurement and analysis of crime and justice: Criminal Justice 2000,* (Vol. 4, pp. 33-83). Washington, DC: National Institute of Justice, Office of Justice Programs.

Tolan, P., Ryan, K., & Jaffe, C. (1988). Adolescents' mental health service use and provider, process, and recipient characteristics. *Journal of Clinical Child Psychology, 17,* 229-236.

Tracy, P. E., & Kempf-Leonard, K. (1996). *Continuity and discontinuity in criminal careers.* New York: Plenum Press.

Tracy, P. E., Wolfgang, M. E., & Figlio, R. M. (1985). *Delinquency in two birth cohorts.* Washington, DC: U.S. Department of Justice, Office of Juvenile Justice and Delinquency Prevention.

Tracy, P. E., Wolfgang, M. E., & Figlio, R. M. (1990). *Delinquency careers in two birth cohorts.* New York: Plenum.

Tremblay, R. E., Masse, B., Perron, D., Le Blanc, M., Schwartzman, A. E., Ledingham, J. E. (1992). Early disruptive behavior, poor school achievement, delinquent behavior, and delinquent personality: Longitudinal analyses. *Journal of Consulting and Clinical Psychology, 60,* 64-72.

Tremblay, R. E., Pagani-Kurtz, L, Masse, L. C., Vitaro, F., & Pihl, R. O. (1995). A bi-modal preventive intervention for disruptive kindergarten boys: Its impact through mid-adolescence. *Journal of Consulting and Clinical Psychology, 63,* 560-568.

U.S. Bureau of Justice Statistics (2006). *Criminal offending statistics.* U.S. Department of Justice, Office of Justice Programs. Retrieved April 4, 2006 from http://www.ojp.usdoj.gov/bjs/crimoff.htm# lifetime

U.S. Department of Health and Human Services (1999). *Mental Health: A report of the Surgeon General.* Rockville, MD: U.S. Department of Health and Human Services.

U.S. Department of Health and Human Services (2000). *Child and adolescent violence research.* Bethesda, MD: National Institute of Mental Health.

U.S. Department of Health and Human Services (2001). *Youth violence: A report to the Surgeon General.* Rockville, MD: U.S. Department of Health and Human Services.

U.S Department of Justice, Federal Bureau of Investigation (1984-2002). *Crime in the United States.* Washington, DC: U.S. Government Printing Office.

U.S Department of Justice, Federal Bureau of Investigation (2007). Retrieved June 14, 2007 from http://www.fbi.gov/ucr/06prelim/index.html

U.S. Department of Justice, Office of Juvenile Justice and Delinquency Prevention (1995). *Guide for implementing the Comprehensive Strategy for Serious, Violent, and Chronic Juvenile Offenders.* Washington, DC: U.S. Government Printing Office.

U.S. President's Commission on Law Enforcement and Administration of Justice (1967). *The challenge of crime in a free society.* Washington, DC: U.S. Government Printing Office.

Van Lang, N. D. J., Ferdinand, R. F., & Verhust, F. C. (2007). Predictors of future depression in early and late adolescence. *Journal of Affective Disorders, 97*, 137-144.

Verhulst, F. C., Eussen, M. L., Berden, G. F., Sanders-Woudstra, J., & Van Der Ende, J. (1993). Pathways of problem behaviors from childhood to adolescence. *Journal of the American Academy of Child Adolescent Psychiatry, 32*, 388-396.

Voeller, K. K. S. (1998). Attention-deficit/hyperactivity disorder: Neurobiological and clinical aspects of attention and disorders of attention. In C.E. Coffey and R.A. Brumback (Eds.), *Textbook of pediatric neuropsychiatry* (pp. 97-145). Washington, DC: American Psychiatric Press.

Wahl, O. (1995). *Media madness: Public images of mental illness.* New Brunswick, NJ: Rutgers University Press.

Walker, J. L., Lahey, B. B., Russo, M. F., Frick, P. J., Christ, M. A. G., McBurnett, K., Loeber, R., Stouthamer-Loeber, M., & Green, S. M. (1991). Anxiety, inhibition, and conduct disorder in children: I. Relations to social impairment. *Journal of the American Academy of Child and Adolescent Psychiatry, 30*, 187-191.

Waschbusch, D. A. (2002). A meta-analytic examination of comorbid hyperactive/impulsive/inattention problems and conduct problems. *Psychological Bulletin, 128*, 118-150.

Waslick, B, & Greenhill, L. (1997). Attention deficit/hyperactivity disorder. In J. M. Wiener (Ed.), *Textbook of child and adolescent psychiatry* (2nd ed, pp. 389-410). Washington, DC: American Psychiatric Press.

Wasserman, G. A., Miller, L. S., & Cothern, L. (2000). *Prevention of serious and violent juvenile offending.* Washington, D.C.: U.S. Department of Justice, Office of Juvenile Justice and Delinquency Prevention.

Webster-Stratton, C. (2000). Oppositional-defiant and conduct-disordered children. In M. Hersen and R.T. Ammerman (Eds.), *Advanced abnormal child psychology* (pp. 387-412). Mahwah, NJ: Lawrence Erlbaum Associates.

West, D. J. (1969). *Present conduct and future delinquency.* London: Heinemann.

West, D. J. (1982). *Delinquency: Its roots, careers and prospects.* London: Heinemann.

West, D. J., & Farrington, D. P. (1973). *Who becomes delinquent?* London: Heinemann.

West, D. J., & Farrington, D. P. (1977). *The delinquent way of life.* London: Heinemann.

Widiger, T. A., & Clark, L. A. (2000). Toward DSM-V and the classification of psychopathology. *Psychological Bulletin, 126*(6), 946-963.

Wolfe, D. A., & Mash, E. J. (2006). Behavioral and emotional problems in adolescents. In D. A. Wolfe and E. J. Mash (Eds.), *Behavioral and emotional disorders in adolescents: Nature, assessment, and treatment* (pp. 3-20). New York: Guilford Press.

Wolfgang, M., Figlio, R. M., & Sellin, T. (1972). *Delinquency in a birth cohort.* Chicago: University of Chicago Press.

Wolfgang, M., Thornberry, T. P., & Figlio, R. M. (1987). *From boy to man, from delinquency to crime.* Chicago: University of Chicago Press.

Wolraich, M. L., Hannah, J. N., Pinnock, T. Y., Baumgaertel, A., & Brown, J. (1996). Comparison of diagnostic criteria for attention-deficit hyperactivity disorder in a countrywide sample. *Journal of the American Academy of Child and Adolescent Psychiatry, 35,* 319-324.

Zimring, F. E., & Hawkins, G. (1997). *Crime is the not the problem: Lethal violence in America.* New York: Oxford University Press.

Zoccolillo, M. (1992). Co-occurrence of conduct disorder and its adult outcomes with depressive and anxiety disorders: A review. *Journal of the American Academy of Child and Adolescent Psychiatry, 31,* 547-556.

Zoccolillo, M. (1993). Gender and the development of conduct disorder. *Development and psychopathology, 5,* 65-78.

Index